T0261219

MINNA ZECHNER, LENA NÄRE,
OLLI KARSIO, ANTERO OLAKIVI,
LIINA SOINTU, HANNA-KAISA HOPPANIA
AND TIINA VAITTINEN

THE POLITICS
OF AILMENT

A New Approach to Care

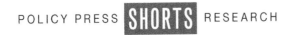

POLICY PRESS **SHORTS** RESEARCH

First published in Great Britain in 2022 by

Policy Press, an imprint of
Bristol University Press
University of Bristol
1-9 Old Park Hill
Bristol
BS2 8BB
UK
t: +44 (0)117 374 6645
e: bup-info@bristol.ac.uk

Details of international sales and distribution partners are available at
policy.bristoluniversitypress.co.uk

British Library Cataloguing in Publication Data
A catalogue record for this book is available from the British Library

ISBN 978-1-4473-4347-9 hardcover
ISBN 978-1-4473-4349-3 ePub
ISBN 978-1-4473-4348-6 ePdf

Cover design: Bristol University Press
Front cover image: iStock/jessicahyde

Policy Press uses environmentally responsible print partners
Printed and bound in Great Britain by CPI Group (UK) Ltd,
Croydon, CR0 4YY

Contents

ONE

Introduction: Humans as ailing beings

At the time of writing this in October 2021, discussions about health, well-being, threat and protection have been all over the media for almost two years. Since 2020, the COVID-19 virus has spread to every continent, infecting over 245 million people (this figure excludes unconfirmed infections) and causing almost five million deaths globally (Coronavirus Resource Center 2021). The impact of the virus on national health care systems, and global and national economies, has been dramatic and continues to be so. While the more privileged countries are vaccinating their populations in an effort to return to international travelling, sports and cultural events, in other parts of the world high numbers of cases are still being witnessed. Notably, public health systems in the global south are on the verge of collapse.

Since the virus crossed from its zoonotic source to humans in 2019, it has affected the entire human population. The epidemic has demonstrated how deeply interconnected human lives are (Springer 2020), and how important it is to approach public health and social care at the interface of the human–animal ecosystem, as is emphasised, for instance, in the One Health approach promoted by the World Health Organization (Hitziger et al 2018), proponents of planetary health (for example Moysés and Soares 2019; Pongsiri et al 2019), and theorists of the eco-welfare state (Gough 2010; 2016; Bailey 2015). The pandemic has also exemplified a key argument of this book: humans are fundamentally interdependent and ailing beings (see also The Care Collective 2020). Acknowledging this as the human condition is a key political and socio-economic issue. According to Michael Fine and Joan Tronto (2020, 307), moreover, the COVID-19 pandemic has demonstrated that 'we can do much to deepen and improve current understanding about care, and of the practices of care and caring, in our world' also in order to safeguard efficient and ethically sustainable responses to future health crises.

The aim of this book is to introduce the concept of ailment as a new theoretical tool for the field of care studies and social sciences more widely. Our concept of ailment begins with the simple realisation that being a body is a bothersome business, and that this fact of life is a starting point for politics and human relatedness. Etymologically, the word ailment comes from the Old English word 'eglan', meaning 'to trouble, plague, afflict' (Merriam-Webster 2021). The word ailment thus refers to the bothering that troubles, afflicts and plagues the body and its embodied mind – and also, as we later argue, larger collectives and societies. Ailment can present itself in different forms, such as minor discomforts that do not go away, extreme pains, or as fears of something troublesome that is constantly present in the background and therefore affects everyday life and demands a response. Ailing individuals need to blow their runny noses. They have sprained ankles that require support bandages or plasters to heal, and they suffer from cancers that demand consuming treatments but may still be deadly. Death as such, and the bothering awareness of the fragility and limits of life, is a source of ailment and actions aiming to alleviate it. The current context of living with a new virus has demonstrated how ailment transforms human lives – inflicting serious illnesses, and creating individual anxiety and global worry that require political action. What troubles the body troubles the mind and vice versa.

The mind is not superior to the body, defining personhood or separating humans from non-humans (Clare 2017).

In addition to ailments in their endless diversity, we use the concept of ailment as an abstract noun. In this sense, ailment is a human condition, or force, that mobilises emotions, actions and relations. As an abstract noun, ailment is about generalised care needs, including the need for self-care, and hence not indicating an immediate dependency on others. While some minor illnesses, or for example a small cut in one's skin, might not consciously bother anybody, they still ail the body, causing it to protect the wound from infection and build the skin anew. Ailment is never only about the individual, however. Rather, ailment is an origin of relatedness that binds human needs together. As we will further elaborate later, ailment takes different forms and manifests in different ailments, bothering all bodies and their embodied minds incessantly. In so doing, ailment produces an innumerable number of (care) needs in the world, as well as prompting responses to those needs. It is in these responses where the relationality and politics of ailment emerge.

The relationality enacted by ailment takes place both within subjects, as well as inter-subjectively. The responses to the ailing of the body and the mind – that is, responses to ailment – may be unconscious responses from within the body-organism itself, for instance when the immune system defends the body against a potentially deadly virus. The responses may also be conscious or unconscious acts of self-care – or self-harm – when the ailing person seeks to alleviate their ailments in different ways. And of course, responses to ailment include active and passive responses to the ailments of others, such as compassion, care, misrecognition and neglect. Contextually, responses to ailment extend from actual concrete encounters between human beings in their immediate environment, to political and institutional responses in societies across the world.

Even if the concept of ailment is defined as generalised care *needs*, and even if some form of care is often the most ethical response to many ailments, it does not mean that responses to ailment are always about care. Virginia Olesen and colleagues (1990, 449) write about 'mundane ailments' that are 'very common, everyday "illnesses" or annoyances, sometimes "ignored" or handled exclusively by the lay person, sometimes brought to the attention of the physician'. In this book, we focus on more serious ailments that are not easily 'ignored' by the ailing person themself, and which, at least potentially, create a need for a response from another person such as a physician, social worker, care worker, family member or another community member. The responses to the needs and ailments of others may be caring, but they may also be neglectful, abusive or in other ways harmful. Tiina Vaittinen (2017) has argued that the varied and innumerable responses to care needs in the world may be imagined as an invisible, constantly changing network of relatedness that organises societies. Similarly, we argue in this book that the innumerable, variant responses to ailment enact a network of relatedness in the world, while at the same time organising societies and their relationships with one another. In these networks, some forms of ailment and some ailing bodies always gain more attention, and more care, than others. That is, some bodies can be deemed as ailing in more powerful ways, capable of mobilising more intense and stickier ailment in the bodies of others – the kind of bothering and troubling that prompts caring responses in other people, as well as in social structures. Simultaneously, the ailments of more marginalised bodies remain invisible, unrecognised and barely responded to by other ways than neglect. As noted by Vaittinen in her theory on the political economies of needs, all bodies are needy and thereby 'the same, yet [they are] never identical in their power to enact relations of care' (Vaittinen 2017, 149). Similarly, while all embodied human beings are ailing, they are differentially powerful in enacting responses that alleviate their ailments. Thus, the politics of ailment emerges in such hierarchies of power.

Furthermore, as two of us (Hoppania and Vaittinen) have written elsewhere, the corporeal character of care relations means that there are latent forces of social disruption at stake in responses to ailment, when mundane situations of inadequate or failed care result in minuscule ruptures, or sometimes in larger systemic changes in the political order. For instance, neglect, inadequate care or violence in care homes for older adults may incite media scandals and politicisation, which then result in the introduction of more or less significant new management practices, monitoring apparatus, or legislative changes. Here, care – as a response to ailment – is 'the political' that forces societies to repeatedly reorder themselves (Hoppania and Vaittinen 2015; Hoppania 2018). We will elaborate this politics of ailment later in this introductory chapter and thereafter examine its operation throughout the book.

In this book we examine the political relatedness that ailment enacts in the world, and the different kinds of social orders that emerge with different personal and collective responses to the needs of ailing subjects. We introduce *homo aegrotus*, the ailing human, who recognises and accepts the physical and mental frailty of all individuals and their ailments. The ailing nature of humans is understood as a permanent and all-encompassing feature that generates action and creates webs of connections in societies. Our concept of ailment contributes to a range of theories relating to care, dependency, debility, dis/ability and vulnerability (for example Noddings 1984; Wærness 1984; Fisher and Tronto 1990; Tronto 1993; 2017; Kittay 1999; Phillips 2007; Fineman 2008; 2010; Mol 2008; Brown 2011; Mackenzie et al 2014; Blackman 2015; Vaittinen 2015; Clare 2017; Puar 2017; Virokannas et al 2018; Engster 2019). Most of the this literature describes the human condition by foregrounding how humans are, for example, vulnerable and dependent on others, and how this vulnerability enacts emotions, actions and relations that follow such a condition. Similarly, ailment directs focus towards 'our dealings with one another' (Spielman 1997, 812), and these dealings include not only care and compassion, but also neglect, ignorance, control and various other ways of responding to ailing bodies and minds.

Vulnerability, dependency, debility and disability can also 'trouble, plague and afflict' individuals and societies. In this sense, vulnerability, dependency, debility, disability and ailment are overlapping concepts. Our conceptualisation of ailment emerges along with writing this book. The book is therefore both an introduction to the concept of ailment and what it can contribute to social theories of care, and a theoretical and scientific exercise where the concept becomes defined, as we think with ailment. Due to the linguistic characteristics of the concept stemming from the verb ail, it offers new possibilities and perspectives. It also offers alternatives to the common, often stigmatising usage of designating entire groups as vulnerable, which renders them as objects of surveillance and regulation (Fineman 2008; Fineman and Grear 2013). Namely, as care theorist Joan Tronto has written, not all relevant concepts already appear within the lexicon of political and social theory, and 'we must expand the terrain to include concepts that are traditionally excluded from politics in order to see how their inclusion changes the contours of political life' (Tronto 2018, 139). One of these concepts is *homines curans*, which carries the notion that humans are essentially caring (Tronto 2017). This understanding resembles *homo aegrotus* in being an alternative way to understand individuals as being different from the calculating, rational and profit-seeking *homo economicus*. However, while *homines curans* emphasises caring as a central human activity, *homo aegrotus* emphasises ailing as inherent in humans – not only are those who receive care ailing, also the caregivers ail.

We believe that the inherently embodied and somewhat old-fashioned, if not biblical concept of ailment – 'to trouble, plague, afflict' – is a term that has been excluded from politics due to its connotations of frailty. We also believe that it should be brought back in, and to the centre of political discourses of care, particularly in ageing societies. In the remainder of this Introduction we pave the way for the thematic chapters of the book by discussing the variety of forms that ailment can take, and briefly returning to what we call the politics of ailment. We then enumerate how and why we *think with* the concept of ailment in the particular context of ageing societies.

On different types of ailment

Ailment as a concept has rarely been explicitly used in research. One of the few texts in which ailment is mentioned is a classic article from 1957 by psychiatrist and psychoanalyst Thomas F. Main. The article, based on a speech given to the British Psychological Society, is entitled 'The Ailment'. It describes the complex relationality of care and emotional labour undertaken by nurses caring for psychiatric patients for whom there was little hope of recovery:

> Whenever something goes wrong with certain distressed patients after lengthy and devoted care, it is not difficult to notice the kind of staff ailment I have described, the same blaming and contempt of others for their limitations of theory, ability, humanity or realism, and the same disclaimers of responsibility. (Main 1957, 141)

The article is based on a study Main conducted in a psychiatric ward. He discovered, for instance, that sedatives would be used in patient care 'only at the moment when she [nurse] had reached the limit of her human resources and was no longer able to stand the patient's problems without anxiety, impatience, guilt, anger or despair' (Main 1957, 130). Administering sedatives helped to ease the worry in the nurses, who became calmer even though it was not they who consumed the sedatives. It was after the nurses recognised that 'ordinary human feelings are inevitable, and they allowed themselves freedom to recognise their negative as well as positive feelings that had hitherto been hidden behind pharmacological traffic' (Main 1957, 130) that the use of sedatives in the ward dropped. A study resembling that of Main was conducted in 2002 by Wendy Gairdner (2002), in which the notion of ailment was used in a similar fashion in relation to the feelings of powerlessness and rivalry that occur in teams that treat children in psychiatric wards.

In Main's study, only certain patients – conceived as special by staff members, together with circumstances in the ward – created what he came to term as 'the ailment'. Main's starting point is in psychiatry and psychoanalysis whereas ours is in the social sciences. But we nevertheless recognise a resemblance between Main's concept of ailment and ours: both emphasise relationality and social dimensions and the effects of illness and caring. In Main's example, ailing patients, that is, their ailing bodies and minds, ail the nurses. Because humans depend on each other, as well as on non-human life, from the moment of conception until death, ailments are never only one's own. As Ron Spielman (1997, 812) notes in his 40th anniversary commentary on Main's article, '[t]he issues [Main] explores in this classic contribution to our literature concern not only patients and staff in psychiatric wards, but all of humanity in our dealings with one another'. Indeed, ailment is the relation that through its bothering effect (ailing) produces care needs and mobilises a variety of direct and indirect responses. Or, as Rozalina V. Ryvkina (2010, 90) puts it, there are social ailments 'whose carrier is not just the human body but also society, social collectives of people'.

Ailment, in other words, is never entirely individualised. It is always already social, relational and, as such, political. This fact is not limited to encounters between patients and nurses. Rather, ailment is a productive force that mobilises emotions and actions, for example to comfort or control, and to mitigate pain and discomfort in ailing beings. Furthermore, it extends from human and non-human beings to entities such as a social community, the maintenance of its welfare and social bonds, or the state of the planetary environment. Sometimes the responses to the ailing subjects' needs are self-care responses; for instance, going to the toilet as a response to the discomforting feeling of 'having to go', or scratching oneself when itchy because of a mosquito bite. At other times, care is needed from other human being(s), for instance in situations where one depends on the help from others in toileting or when itchy because of a mosquito bite. As generalised care needs, the concept of ailment thus goes beyond questions of in/dependency. Care is broadly understood here as those activities that meet the physical, social, psychological and emotional needs and requirements of another living being (for example Tronto 1993).

The concept of ailment foregrounds that, under all circumstances, also those who give care or do care work are ailing; psychologically as the studies by Main (1957) and Gairdner (2002) demonstrate, as well as physically, if not because of the workload, for the sheer reason that such carers are embodied living organisms. In care research, the tension between the needs of care receiver and carer have remained difficult to address simultaneously (for example Kittay 2005; Simplican 2015; Vaittinen 2019). It has been difficult to consider the vulnerability of both parties in the care relationship without blaming or neglecting one or the other party. For example, some parents with disabilities feel pathologised when some studies assume that their impairments are seriously affecting the well-being and development of their children and making them, by default, (young) carers to their parents (Newman 2002, 620). The concept of ailment thus provides a view that escapes the dualities that are often present in our thinking about care – ailment brings subjects together, but it can do so in surprising, unpredictable and non-linear ways, as we demonstrate throughout the book.

Political responses to ailment

Ailment is a relational force that requires responses and mobilises politics. The concept of ailment emphasises active effects and chains of embodied reactions: the relationality of ailing subjects. We argue that ailment, understood as a political concept, can provide a concept from which to think of agency, resistance and solidarity stemming from the ailing human condition. This perspective does not reduce the agency of ailing subjects, rather, it expands the realms of agency (cf Barad 2007). Indeed, human ailments should be seen as agentive: irrespective of people's will, they produce effects and affects. They constrain, as well as force, bodies and minds to react. Ailment operates as a relational force that evokes and elicits responses such as anxiety, helplessness, disgust and horror, but also tenderness and a sense of responsibility, as well as practical, organisational and institutional responses such as practices of caring or neglect, solidary relations and grass-roots organisation, economic and social policies, and business activities. What remains constant in these various responses is the productivity of ailment.

Denial and ignorance can be collective responses to ailment as well. Complete and permanent denial and ignorance are difficult, however, since ailment tends to trouble and bother societies regardless of whether these societies explicitly acknowledge and recognise it. Some level of care is always necessary for the survival of any community. As an example, one can consider the global vaccination politics surrounding the COVID-19 pandemic. The hoarding of vaccines in richer parts of the world, combined with the political decision to protect the intellectual property rights of the vaccine-producing companies, has led to an uneven distribution of protection against the virus globally, with rising death tolls seen particularly in the majority world. But the virus and its new variants will remain a global health threat until it is contained by vaccines also in the majority world. This example underlines the inevitable entanglement of humans with one another and their environment, as ignoring and neglecting the ailments of the poorer populations will end up ailing the richer ones as well. Richer countries can try to ignore these ailments, but living in denial is hardly a sustainable, long-term solution to a global pandemic.

Even in the most ethical politics of ailment, some ailments can be, and must be, left without political attention, for the sheer reason that it is practically impossible to care about all possible ailments in the world simultaneously: that is, responding to some ailments will always mean disregarding others (Vaittinen 2017). With the *politics of ailment*, we refer to the decisions regarding which kinds of ailments, and whose ailments, are understood as worthy of political attention, and where collective responses to comfort ailing beings are deemed as necessary; which ailments are knowingly left without attention; and which, further still, are not even noticed in the prevailing system of politics. The call for such explicit political discussions of ailment is one of the main aims of this book (see also Hoppania et al 2016). Such debates, and the related debates on the distribution of economic resources among the ailing, are often actively avoided in daily politics, which tends to avoid decisions 'about who in fact provides care, who pays for it (and how much), who does the labour, gets paid or does not get paid for it, who receives care and who might be neglected?' (Hoppania 2015, 165).

Responses to ailment draw on a variety of cultural assumptions regarding the value and deservingness of different groups and individuals. When facing the ailments of distant and marginalised others, people and societies can employ self-comforting discourses to explain and justify neglect and inaction. When others are societally misrecognised as non-deserving or responsible for their own well-being, their ailments are also misrecognised as private matters rather than collective problems. Their ailments do not ail and bother others (affectively and emotionally) as much as the ailments of people who are categorised as deserving. Thus, practices of misrecognition can work like the mollifying sedatives featured in Main's (1957) example. The ailments of marginalised others may even be interpreted against the group's best interest when connected to societal power hierarchies and ideologies, such as racism. For example, when slavery was abolished in the United States, hundreds of thousands of African Americans died of preventable diseases due to poverty and a lack of adequate housing and health care. But their overrepresentation in the casualties of smallpox was interpreted by dominant racist society as nature's way of getting rid of people who were not suited for freedom (Downs 2012, 103). The ailment of African Americans was understood to reflect their inferiority in the societal and biological hierarchies, which then led to the dangerous and unjust outcome of not providing means to tackle the smallpox virus.

As Spielman (1997, 812) notes, ailment is not only ' "an acute specific disease" but something harder to define, something pervasive (insidious, perhaps) yet debilitating and causing distress'. Here, the operation of ailment bears resemblance to affects as being inherently 'sticky'. Ailment, like affect, sticks to human bodies and impacts social systems (cf Ahmed 2004a; 2004b). Ailment clearly has an affective dimension. In a strong sense, ailing subjects create affective relations. When faced with actualised ailments of loved ones, people tend to feel a sense of responsibility urging them to act and respond (for example Sointu 2018). At the same time, ailing subjects can mobilise affects of danger, repulsion, even disgust, as seen in the wards that Main examined. In her study on nurses working on a ward for burns victims, Trudy Rudge (2009, 240) noticed how nurses described the emotion work that they undertook to overcome the initial horror they felt around severely burned patients. These nurses were met with both fear and admiration by nurses working on other wards (Rudge 2009, 241).

According to Sara Ahmed, affects do things and align individuals and communities through the very intensity of their attachments. Affects are thus not solemnly subjective experiences. Instead, they 'mediate the relationship between the psychic and the social, and between the individual and the collective' (Ahmed 2004a, 119). Ailment evoking affects both within ailing bodies and minds, as well as other bodies and minds exposed to the ailing of others, does things and binds subjects together. Ailment involves subjects and objects and leaves a trace (cf Ahmed 2004a, 119). Even though everyone ails, the ailment of certain groups has always been affectively stickier and politically more difficult to ignore than the ailment of others. Moreover, social hierarchies related to ailment also concern those who are given the task to attend to the ailment of others, as we discuss in Chapter four in particular.

Thinking with ailment in an ageing world

If the demographic revolution of the past century was rapid population growth due to increasing fertility and a decline in mortality, we are currently witnessing a phase in the demographic revolution of population ageing due to declining fertility and increased longevity. The share of over-60-year-olds in the world population more than doubled from 1980 to 2017 and is expected to double again by 2050 (UN 2017). Hence, the question of how to respond to the increasing needs for care in ageing societies is a crucial backdrop for the politics of ailment, as we develop in this book. While our empirical examples stem from developed welfare states, the concept of ailment is by no means limited to them. The conceptual lens of ailment makes visible that ageing and responding to its consequences concern the whole of society, and consequently engender new relations between individuals, groups and institutions.

We suggest the concept of ailment as a concept and tool to *think with* the past and the future of ageing societies (see also de la Bellacasa 2012). Drawing on Donna Haraway, María Puig de la Bellacasa (2012) argues against the individualised notion of thinking and knowing, proposing the idea of thinking and knowing as relational and collective processes. In this book, we think with ailment in two distinct ways. First, we use ailment as a concept to 'think-with' and ask how the world, and particular the ageing societies within it, can be understood as being built through responses to ailment. Second, in this book our method of working has been a collective 'thinking-with'.

The book is the outcome of a collective process of thinking and writing together that began in 2013, when we established our Viva collective. We come from different disciplinary backgrounds in Sociology, Social Policy, Political Science, International Relations, Peace Research, and Global Health, but have all conducted research on elder care. Individually, we have been conducting empirical research on ageing, social and care policies and politics, daily practices of elder care and nursing, informal spousal care, management of elder care work, migrant elder care and domestic workers, globally recruited nurses, and the financialisation and marketisation of care, to name some examples (Anttonen and Zechner 2011; Karsio and Anttonen 2013; Vaittinen 2014, 2015, 2017, 2019; Hoppania 2015; 2018; Hoppania and Vaittinen 2015; Olakivi 2017; Sointu 2018; Näre and Diatlova 2020; Morgan and Zechner 2022; Näre and Cleland Silva 2021; Olakivi and Wrede 2021; Sointu et al 2021; Zechner 2022).

In spring 2013 we were frustrated with how Finnish elder care policies and politics had forgotten ailment, and instead portrayed the objects of those policies as free, unencumbered individuals able to make rational choices on care service markets. To participate in these political debates and discussions, we decided to establish a research collective that we named Viva, referring both to viva voce, the oral examination that characterises our way of working on our ideas through discussion and debate, but also to Viva! as a salute but also an exclamation for 'long live!', as we do while ailing. Finally, the pronunciation of viva in English as /ˈvʌɪvə/ is similar to *vaiva*, the Finnish word for ailment, and the Finnish name of the collective (Vaivakollektiivi).

Our debates and discussions led to a co-authored book in Finnish entitled *Hoivan Arvoiset. Vaiva yhteiskunnan ytimessä*, that is, 'Worthy of care – Ailment in the heart of society'

(Hoppania et al 2016). In the present book we seek to translate the politics of ailment from the Finnish language and discourse of *vaivapolitiikka* into a discourse and politics that resonates also in other contexts, internationally. The Finnish monograph serves as a basis for this book, but we have developed our thinking on ailment further and rewritten our argument with an international readership in mind. Since the publication of *Worthy of Care*, we have as a collective contributed to debates on management in elder care (Hoppania et al 2021), intersectional inequalities in older age and care (Karsio et al 2020), marketisation and privatisation of care services (Vaittinen et al 2018) and the financialisation of elder care (Hoppania et al 2022).

The following thematic chapters illustrate the ways in which ailment operates as a productive force in society, and the multifaceted consequences that derive from ailment as a central human condition. Our aim is to think of the past and present of social policies and elder care with and through the concept of ailment, thereby describing *what ailment does* in and for the world. In Chapter two we provide a historical perspective on the development of social policies as collective responses to ailment from pre-modern times in Europe to the emergence of contemporary advanced welfare states. Chapter two demonstrates that human ailment has always provided societal responses and reactions, and that contemporary welfare states are simply much more complicated and advanced forms of those collective responses. We also discuss the ways in which responses to ailment are, and have from early on been, characterised by elements of care as well as of control, exploitation and profit making.

In Chapter three we offer an analysis on key current trends of marketisation and financialisation of care as neoliberal responses to ailment. Neoliberalism is here understood as an ideological and political project of reorganising international capitalism to enhance conditions for capital accumulation and to restore the power of economic elites (Harvey 2005). Neoliberal politics has advanced the commodification, marketisation and financialisation of elder care, for instance by introducing market mechanisms into the realm of public care provision (for example Brennan et al 2012; Dahl 2017; Zechner 2022) and allowing the financial engineering of corporate profits in marketised care (Horton 2022; Hoppania et al 2022). The third chapter demonstrates that one way in which ailment's productivity appears in society is through the generation of new markets and financial activities and devices. The central paradox that we highlight is that while ailment creates new business opportunities, the neoliberal discourse nevertheless continues to conceive ageing as a burden for national economies. Hence, neoliberal responses to ailment remain inadequate because they fail to acknowledge the nature of ailment as unpredictable and changing from one day to the next similarly to care, and thus impossible to commodify in any simplistic way.

Chapter four focuses on care relations and demonstrates how ailment mobilises concrete, embodied and emotional responses in immediate social encounters, along with gendered, racialised and classed divisions of labour that extend to the global scale. We introduce the notion of caregiver ailment to emphasise the relationality and affective qualities of ailment in the daily practices of attending to ailment. Finally, the concluding chapter develops the concept of the politics of ailment further and explores its usability also in relation to climate change and the economic recovery after the pandemic.

TWO

Tracing ailment in social and care policies

Throughout human history, individuals, households and communities have responded to ailment in their everyday practices. Human remains from Ancient Greece, for example, show that people with illnesses, chronic conditions, and developmental defects were provided with care (Dasen 2015). Ailing bodies, especially the bodies of the elites, have thus mobilised social action. Written evidence from medieval Europe tells the same story (Kuuliala 2015), and along with individuals and private households, there have been joint social efforts to respond to ailment, in accordance with the contemporary ethical standards and resources (see, for example, Reich 1995). Churches, local communities, and states have made various efforts to keep people alive. However, neglect, control and abuse have also been common responses to ailment. People have died – and continue to die – due to a lack of appropriate treatment, sustenance, accommodation and care. Control, exploitation and the benefiting from other people's ailments are also part of the history of care and social policy.

In this chapter, we focus on how ailment as a social force has historically manifested itself in social and care policies. Through our exploration, we demonstrate how ailment creates specific relations and responses, and how these responses combine elements of care, control and profit making in different degrees depending on the historical, political and social contexts. We propose that the concept of ailment opens new perspectives on the history of care. On the one hand, ailment encompasses the various illnesses and afflictions that anybody may experience. On the other hand, it refers to the existential relationality stemming from the ailments encountered by all individuals – that is, the political and social processes that the ailing condition produces and mobilises. Albeit stemming from the bodies and minds of individuals, ailment is never entirely individualised. It is always already social, relational and political. Since ailment is sticky and affects not only the ailing individuals but also others around them, collective responses have been created as responses to various ailments. This makes ailment a mobilising force for social policies. When redistributing wealth and accumulating health and well-being, social policies are ways to address ailment.

In emphasising the significance of relationality, interdependence and collective responses, our thinking is in line with many existing theories of care (Kittay 2005; Tronto 2017). There is, however, a slight shift in perspective when we look at the history of care and social policy departing from the ailing human being, *homo aegrotus*, instead of care and *homines curans* (Tronto 2017; see Chapter one). Human societies are not always or completely caring in their responses to human neediness, and domination and oppression may at times be embedded even within care itself. This darker side of care has of course been acknowledged by several care and disability researchers before us (see, for example, Tronto 1993, 109; Simplican 2015; Clare 2017; Kelly 2017). But through our focus on ailment – instead of care provision itself – we are able to further illuminate the complexity of responses and relations in care.

The value of human life and the responses to ailment have varied: those with more resources have had better access to care and other forms of support. One response to these inequalities has been the welfare state, where resources are collected and pooled to respond to various human needs (Titmuss 1974; Esping-Andersen 1985; Briggs 2006). Even though expanding welfare states responded to ailment more extensively than previous societal arrangements, inequality, exploitation and exclusion are embedded in the historical structures of welfare states – both within nations states and globally. Like other societal responses to ailment, welfare states are equally part of the relations and dynamics ailment produces in the world. Despite the vast support and services the welfare state provides for ailing individuals, it also controls and governs human ailment.

Social policies also always draw boundaries that define whose ailments are addressed, how, and on what grounds (for instance, who is eligible for care and for what kind of care), and which groups and which kinds of ailments can be left without a collective caring response. This chapter demonstrates, through various historical and present-day examples, how ailment has driven certain kinds of responses, and social and care policies; how ailment has been addressed in these policies; and how care intersects with control, exploitation and profit making. As illustrative examples, we discuss how three distinct welfare states, namely the United Kingdom, Finland and Germany, have evolved in their responses to ailment.

Social policies have mainly tackled social or economic problems, and they have not explicitly acknowledged and recognised ailment as a mobilising force and a shared human condition. Implicitly, however, European social policies have addressed ailment in various ways, albeit mainly in subordination to more powerful interests, including economic interests. Societal changes, such as industrialisation, have created the need to address issues, such as care, which used to belong to the private sphere of life at a public policy level. Industrialisation increasingly moved work and production from households to factories and cities, and children and older adults in need of care at home could not be attended to while working. The care of older adults has relatively lately become an explicit target for policies, but early social policies, while predominantly addressing the problems of poverty, also responded at least partially to what we call ailment.

We have divided the history of social and care policies into four periods, which loosely follow the development of social policies and the western welfare state. First, we investigate responses to ailment through sanctions in the era before the Bismarckian social policy reform in Prussia and Imperial Germany, and Beveridgean social policy in the United Kingdom, which are typically defined as the beginnings of modern social policy. Second, we focus on the period from the late 19th century until the end of the Second World War, when social policy arrangements focused especially on reproducing the workforce. Then we proceed to the rise of the modern welfare state and the expansion of social rights: a period when caring responses to ailment were rather extensive, at least in the Nordic countries. Towards the end of this chapter, we shift our focus to care policies, since care has become a central social policy issue and is an essential response to ailment. Finally, we examine how the social and care policies of the new millennium have responded and continue to respond to ailment, when permanent austerity politics, global free markets and the foregrounding of personal responsibility dominate the collective responses in social politics.

Sanctioning the ailing

One obvious way that early European social policies responded to ailment was through poverty relief and the poorhouse system. Poorhouses (also called almshouses, workhouses, poor-farms, or city homes) were institutions that housed the poor and those who lacked accommodation. These included, for example, people with disabilities or mental or physical illnesses, children without custodians, and older adults, and they were obliged to work in exchange for assistance. The poorhouses were generally local arrangements (Hitchcock 1985; Anttonen and Sipilä 2000), but often based on poor laws governing populations and the labour force in societies where large proportions of the population were living in poverty. The first Poor Law in England was enacted in 1388 to deal with the labour shortage after the Black Death, and in 1601 the Elizabethan Poor Law established local areas' responsibility for the poor who were old or sick (Greve 2014, 4).

In Finland as well, a poorhouse system was established in the 14th century. Later, in the 19th century, following the New Poor Law in England and Wales in 1834 and in Finland in 1879, poorhouses began to develop clear disciplinary aims and were generally reserved for the unproductive poor, meaning those who would have been able to work, but for various reasons did not. The workhouses were correctional institutions for the poor, who were defined as undeserving (Wagner 2005, 4–6). The workhouse system is thus an early example of how material responses to human ailment coexist with the practices through which humans are categorised, for example, as 'deserving' and 'undeserving'. These categorisations are always entangled in broader socio-technical responses to various ailments. Due to politically produced and institutionalised categorisation systems and the affects they mobilise, people can conceive it as both natural and justified that some ailments are responded to with care, others with neglect and ignorance, and yet others with correction, punishment and sanctioning, as in the case of the workhouse system. In these political configurations, the societal responses to ailment can also be disciplining and seen as governmentalising moves in the Foucauldian sense of the term.

One reason for setting up the poorhouse system was the unrest that people who were conceived of, and categorised as, 'loitering people', who were unable or unwilling to cater for themselves, were considered to create in society (Anttonen and Sipilä 2000). Physical ailment manifested in a lack of food and shelter of the populations living in poverty was disturbing, in other words 'ailing' the better-off populations who witnessed the sickness, dirt and unrest of those in poverty. The physical ailment of those living in poverty created thus a more psychological, moral and affective ailment to the elites, in a similar manner as with Main's (1957) study of the nurses in psychiatric wards whose patients did not progress despite their treatment. Similar to the nurses who administered sedatives to ease their own worry, the members of the higher strata in society also administered support to help people in poverty at least partly in order to ease their own distress caused by ailment. The isolation of people from the public space to poorhouses and workhouses, where they would be less visible, can also be seen as a way for the elites to alleviate their own negative affects – that is, their ailment in the sense of 'troubling', 'bothering' and 'annoying' – caused by the need to encounter suffering, pain, sickness and dirt in their own daily environment.

Management in the form of assistance, punishment and isolation of the ailing poor thus served various purposes – ranging from disciplining the poor to offering psychological, moral and affective alleviation to the elite – and so became more organised as the wealth of nations accumulated. It also helped to create societal harmony and to ensure the supply of labour. The idea behind English poorhouses was also to boost the morale of the nation: the idle masses would be replaced by hard-working labourers (Hitchcock 1985, 5). In 18th-century Finland, care for the poor was mainly the responsibility of the parishes. The main criteria for inclusion were that the poor people had no family or friends to care for them, and that they were not able to work due to illness (Miettinen 2018, 295–9). From the 19th century onwards, those without accommodation, family and basic sustenance were sold by the parishes and later by municipalities to households that offered to provide basic sustenance for the lowest price – often in exchange for work (Karisto et al 1988, 129–30; Kröger et al 2003, 28; Halmekoski 2011).

The workhouse reforms which took place in the 19th century marked a change in public attitudes towards the poor. Even though the entire poorhouse and workhouse system represents a sanctioning response to ailment, the new 19th-century workhouses, in particular, conceived the ailing individuals as personally flawed and responsible for their condition. The idea of putting all the capable poor to work was thus emphasised (Annola 2019). The poor and ailing either worked in the workhouses or, if capable, in a 'real job' outside the workhouse. The old poorhouses and existing workhouses were in some cases merely unattended dwellings provided by the parishes or municipalities. The poor laws, both in the United Kingdom and in Finland, also restricted the mobility of those in custody (Crowther 1981/2016; Luttinen 2019), thus managing the supply of the workforce geographically. This management function became even more significant with increasing industrialisation and urbanisation. The working conditions in the factories were often dangerous, and factory owners were obliged to provide sustenance for individuals who had lost their ability to work due to working in their factory. The poor laws, however, provided an opportunity for factory owners to reduce their financial responsibility since the 1852 Poor Law in Finland made everyone not able to provide for themselves entitled to public relief (see Voionmaa 1929, 404). In addition, the poor laws provided a moral opportunity for factory owners to use child labour, and by 'providing work' for children, they proved to play their part in alleviating poverty, which was good news for municipalities (Voionmaa 1929, 406–7).

Similar to factories, the conditions in poorhouses were harsh. Those residing there were expected to work for their maintenance. Inmates also lost their political rights (Marshall 1950, 33). This happened as late as the beginning of the 20th century in Finland, where women had been granted the right to vote on equal terms with men in 1906. In the 1911 Finnish elections, several voters, especially women and older adults, lost their right to vote because they were receiving poor relief

(Einiö et al 2018). Thus, the harsh conditions served as a message not to become an inmate unless there was no other choice. This is a telling example of the political implications of sanctioning the ailing in society, where certain groups of ailing individuals were penalised by reducing their citizenship rights.

Similarly in the United Kingdom, the early modern social policies contained elements of sanctioning and governing the ailing. Social policy scholars have traced the beginnings of modern social policy to the poorhouse system, or more specifically to the debate following the Speenhamland Law to Poor Laws Reform in 1834 in the United Kingdom (Gough 2008, 39; Béland and Mahon 2016, 5–6). This is mainly because of the connection between the rise of free market capitalism and early forms of social protection in association with managing the labour force. Daniel Béland and Rianne Mahon (2016, 5–7) discuss the relationship between market capitalism and the rise of early social policy, drawing from Karl Polanyi's take on the English Poor Law debate after the Speenhamland Law (1795). This law set limits to free market capitalism by requiring that the state guarantees a minimum income for the poor. The law contributed to more extensive poor relief outside the poorhouses, but the system was seen by advocators of free markets to harm economic progress by decreasing the supply of 'free labour'. After a long debate, the Speenhamland Law, including the outdoor relief system, was abolished by the Poor Law Reform in 1834. This contributed to the punitive and stigmatising aspect of social assistance, targeted only at those 'weaklings' (Marshall 1950, 32) who had absolutely no option but to enter a poorhouse (Béland and Mahon 2016, 5–6, 13; see also Marshall 1950, 32–3).

The poorhouse and workhouse systems represent forms of early social policies, but they can also be understood as 'an embryonic social service' (Crowther 1981/2016, 269). This is partly because workhouses gradually began to provide hospital treatment in areas of the United Kingdom that otherwise lacked such facilities. The system also provided asylum for the needy: those who were chronically ill, without families and unable to support themselves or whose ailments were not responded to by other, more primary means. In the 1900s, the poverty relief system became incorporated into the gradually developing welfare systems and their new ways of responding to ailment. With the development of modern welfare states, rising life expectancy and rising standards of living, the ailments of older adults began to be perceived as part of the public responsibility. This politicisation of the ailment of older populations happened both in the United Kingdom and in Finland (Crowther 1981/2016, 269; Anttonen and Sipilä 2000). But despite a long time having passed from the days of the poorhouse, public elder care institutions still carry a stigmatising label in the minds of many, especially among older adults.

From the perspective of ailment, this long period of poorhouses and workhouses represents the birth of the idea that societies could, and maybe even should, organise collective responses to human ailment because it is beneficial for all of society. Thus, even though ailing people were mostly penalised for their troubles, the seeds of modern and organised social policy had been planted.

Protecting the ailing workforce

As the example of poorhouses demonstrates, employment and social policies were interconnected from early on. Before wider, national social policy systems were created to ensure workforce availability, smaller-scale arrangements were organised in many countries around factories. Taking care of certain ailments of their employees and their families (for example housing needs, hygiene, adequate nutrition) provided factories with a fit and competent workforce, but also protected the wider community from other ailments such as communicable diseases. Some factory owners provided basic education, health and social care, and sometimes also accommodation, for the workers and their families (Anttonen and Sipilä 2000; Reckendrees 2020). These exclusive and limited social policy solutions in factory communities were a result of industrialisation and urbanisation. As national systems did not yet exist, the patrons and workers came up with arrangements of their own. Ailment of workers, along with local arrangements in parishes in the countryside, was perhaps the first push towards an acknowledgement and recognition of ailment at the societal level. Responding to human ailment was no longer seen as only a private and a moral and religious-ethical issue and a question of offering affective and psychological comfort to the elites; instead, it had to do with the wealth of the nations as well. In the late 19th century, the first national social policy systems were created in Prussia (Beck 1997).

In the 1880s Chancellor Otto von Bismarck introduced the social insurance, sickness, accident, old-age and invalidity legislation in Germany, motivated by keeping the workers satisfied and less occupied with socialist activities (Bonoli 1997). The most skilled, politically active, and educated workers had already become organised before social insurance legislation, and the need to protect the workers was recognised not only by workers, but also by employers. Skilled and organised workers had negotiating power and could thus make claims regarding their protection. Or, following our argument about ailment as a social force: since these workers recognised their proneness to different kinds of ailments and their consequences for their abilities to work, they mobilised and were able to mobilise for protection. While workers in the United States relied on market-based insurance, the continental European countries preferred to rely on collective occupational social insurance funds administered by the representatives of employees and employers, which sought to stay independent from the state (Palier 2010, 36).

Bismarckian social policies were based on social insurance that provided earnings-related benefits, disability and accident insurance, and free medical care for male employees.

Entitlements were conditional on contribution, and financing was mainly based on employer or employee contributions (Fay 1950). Social welfare institutions supplemented the economy, and merit, work performance and productivity were required to receive social assistance (Titmuss 1974, 31). The system further created hierarchies in addressing ailment. The clientele of social security was divided into administrative categories, defined, for example, as workers in heavy industry, production of consumer goods, or agriculture (Fuchs and Offe 2009). The care needs of children, women and older adults, or the wider context of ailing, were not explicitly addressed, but by ensuring the income levels of male workers even in the case of unemployment and injury, the dependents' income was at least to some extent looked after as well. Accident pensions even included higher additional payments for the benefit of children, grandchildren, parents and grandparents (Fay 1950). However, those without a provider needed to rely on the church. From the perspective of ailment, the Bismarckian social policies focused on male breadwinners, thus making those not in paid employment directly dependent on them. This demonstrates that the ailments of working males were defined as worthy of protection, whereas the ailments of women and children were not as closely attended to.

In contrast to the Bismarckian approach focusing on workers, the British Beveridgean social policy aimed at the prevention of poverty in general (Bonoli 1997). At the time of the Second World War, the British early unemployment insurance system from 1911 was criticised for having the same qualities that the Bismarckian social insurance was based on: namely a great variety in different provisions for sickness and disability, and their relationship to other social security provisions (Abel-Smith 1992, 4). A committee was set up to address these questions in 1941 and the economist William Beveridge prepared a report with the insight that social welfare needs to be conjoined with economic policy. The aim was full employment. After the Second World War the economy was booming, and full employment was attainable. However, Beveridge's approach was different from Bismarck's since he suggested that social security could cover the entire nation, not just those who were working. Another radical suggestion was that health care would be made available to everybody (Beveridge 1942). The benefit levels in Beveridgean social policy were characterised by universal provision, entitlement was based on residence or need, and benefits were typically flat-rate and financed through general taxation. The underlying understanding of ailment in the Beveridgean approach was that it concerned everybody: all individuals, or at least citizens, were seen as potentially ailing, and their ailments were seen as potentially ailing (that is, bothering) the well-being and prosperity of other citizens. Those with similar ailments were considered equal in the sense that they were allotted the same level of benefit across social strata. However, the Beveridgean model still relied heavily on the male-breadwinner model, thus making those who were not in salaried employment (women) still dependent on those who worked (able-bodied men) (Powell and Hewitt 2002).

In sum, both the Bismarckian and the Beveridgean social policies aimed at securing the labour market workforce and at the reproduction of citizens, but the methods were merely defined differently. The Bismarckian approach focused on the workforce and therefore left most women, children and other individuals not in employment outside social policy measures. Despite its heavy reliance on the male-breadwinner model, the Beveridgean approach of securing the workforce also recognised women as part of the public social policy measures, and therefore opened the door for wider public responsibility for ailment and care.

Despite these differences, both Bismarckian and Beveridgean social policies can be interpreted as establishing the idea that human ailment is worthy of collective attention and security. This was manifested as the awareness of risks, to both individuals and collectives, of illness or disability, which can lead to loss of livelihood and thus threaten the social, political, economic and moral order of society. Human ailment, if left unattended, was coming to be understood as harmful for workers, employers and the whole of society – and also as posing a political threat: if the workers would not comply with the dominant social, political and economic order, this would create room for other orders, such as socialism. As a response to all of these issues, legislation and institutions of provision and financing (such as insurance) were created to provide security for the risk of being unable to work due to illness, old age and disability.

Acknowledging ailment

After the Second World War ended and populations began to grow, new political winds began to blow. The value of human life was replenished, and in many countries social policies were planned to support people based on social rights, at least to an extent that had never been seen before. This meant, in many ways, the birth of the welfare state in its modern sense. Different paths led to different outcomes. In terms of social policy, Bismarckian social policy developed into a conservative model which is dominant in Central Europe, whereas Beveridgean social policy developed into two models. The liberal model of Beveridgean universalistic social policy was developed in Britain, and a social democratic model was developed in the Nordic countries (Esping-Andersen 1990).

Esping-Andersen's (1990) classic work divides welfare states into three worlds of welfare capitalism: Conservative, Liberal, and Social Democratic. The liberal welfare states offer a minimal provision of welfare, benefits are modest, and often the entitlement criteria are strict, with recipients usually being means tested and being a beneficiary seen as stigmatising. In the conservative welfare state, benefits are often earnings related, administered through the employer, and geared towards maintaining existing social patterns. The role of the family is also emphasised. In the social democratic welfare state, welfare provision is characterised by universal and comparatively generous benefits. There is a strong commitment to full employment and income protection, and the state has a strong role in promoting equality through a redistributive social security system.

This well-known division, we argue, can be understood as a division between different ways to acknowledge and govern human ailment in modern societies. The three models are not only political responses to individual vulnerabilities, but they are also and primarily political responses to the ability of ailing beings to ail other ailing beings. It is the ability of an ailing person to ail others and the wider society – that is, the bothering aspect of ailment – that these models aim to recognise and govern through their different ways and forms. Despite the differences in the form, coverage or level of social protection in different welfare states, they all mark a significant improvement in acknowledging basic human needs as an essential part of citizenship (Anttonen et al 2012). In the course of time, welfare state policies extended across various ailments to cover livelihoods during sickness, old age and unemployment, as well as health and social care.

By the 2020s, various care and welfare needs emerging from ailment have come to be recognised as worthy of public recognition and support. A steep increase has emerged in public social expenditure as a share of gross domestic product since the 1880s in the western world. The expansion of public social expenditure began after the Second World War, but in many countries the share has doubled since the 1960s (Ortiz-Ospina and Roser 2016). The expansive welfare state is thus a relatively recent phenomenon.

As mentioned earlier, the poor laws before the time of welfare states often deprived citizens of their civil rights. With the development of social insurance in the late 19th century, the rights of citizens began to expand to social rights and social citizenship, as termed by Marshall (1950). When legislated social rights are established, the importance of family, philanthropy and markets in responding to ailment decreases. The basis of distribution in these areas is shifted from individual resources and market power to political actors (Esping-Andersen 1985; Korpi 1989, 313). The welfare state that, after the Second World War, was in many European countries based on linking economic policy, economic growth, and the welfare state, has been called the Keynesian welfare state (Kuusi 1964). Here, policies aimed to create active markets and growth, while also controlling them. The surplus created and partly collected by taxes and other social contributions allowed for the extension of welfare state programmes. Claims on those welfare state programmes were not extensive due to economic growth (Offe 1983). Thus, economic growth made it possible to expand social rights and responses to ailment, but they depend on continuous economic growth, which, if based on the use of non-renewable resources, is destined to end at some point. The dependency of welfare state programmes on economic growth also contributes to new ailments, such as ecological and social crises caused by climate change.

The realisation of social rights has taken various forms in the different welfare states. In the Central European model, family has shouldered the main responsibility for care. The idea of subsidiarity is strong; and only when families and communities cannot take care of their members does the state or public authority intervene. As an example of the liberal welfare state, the United Kingdom historically had a strong expanding welfare state that emphasised the social rights aspect after the Second World War. Until the end of the 1970s, when Margaret Thatcher and the Conservatives took power, most means-tested social services were publicly provided, and, for example, a strong public housing system existed. Thatcher's era launched a massive wave of privatisation and marketisation (see Chapter three) of the public sector and social services. As the care services were mainly means tested, the change was not as drastic in the care sector as it was in housing services or public transport. Nevertheless, over the succeeding decades, the social services were outsourced, and citizens transformed from service receivers into active citizen-consumers with free choice and personal budgets for arranging care (Clarke 2006; Clarke et al 2007). We will return to this in the following chapter.

While the liberal welfare state was developed towards individual and market reliance in service provision, the social democratic welfare state was geared towards dependence on state and public authorities. In long-term care policies, at the legislative level, this meant that the responsibility for care was explicitly shifted from families to public authorities. That is, care became a social right, and, at least formally, it still is (Anttonen and Karsio 2017). Although families continue to play a significant role in providing informal care (Van Aerschot 2014), local authorities (municipalities) were assigned the practical and legal responsibility for providing care. The universalistic welfare state began to develop rapidly after the Second World War and gradually expanded to offer considerable public coverage of social protection through benefits and services that were targeted at the entire population, according to need. Social security (pensions, unemployment benefits and sickness benefits), and health and social services were aimed to cover all citizens instead of being granted as means-tested social assistance for those most in need (as in the liberal model), or as benefits based on employment status (as in the conservative model) (Anttonen and Sipilä 2000). As such, the social democratic welfare state meant increasing the recognition of ailment as part of human life across all social classes.

Consequently, a solid infrastructure for health and social service delivery was built. Universal provision of services and benefits meant that everyone is entitled to social protection on the basis of residence. Old age homes and home care services became part of the municipal care service system. In Norway and Sweden, and also in Finland, the 1950s and 1960s witnessed the birth of the personalised universal elder care service system

(Vabø and Szebehely 2012, 124). The origins of home care services lay particularly in the third sector, where civil society organisations operated. Their services were included and organised under municipalities and became part of the tax-based system (Anttonen and Sipilä 2000). Home care services, in particular, meant freedom for older adults from having to rely on family or moving to an old age home, which – at the time – still carried the stigma of the poorhouse (Anttonen and Sipilä 2000; Vabø and Szebehely 2012, 124). Women continued to have the primary responsibility for responding to ailment through care. For many women, however, the expansion of the public system enabled increasing economic independence and novel opportunities for stable employment and professionalisation in paid care work (Wrede et al 2008). Simultaneously, the Nordic labour markets became highly segregated, a condition that still prevails (for example Kauhanen and Riukula 2019). Consequently, women have been the main sufferers of the later devaluation of paid care in the Nordic countries (Wrede et al 2008; Hansen et al 2021), as we discuss in Chapter four.

A central way in which welfare states respond to ailment is by developing long-term care. For example, in Germany ailment is recognised through compulsory long-term care insurance, and the vast majority (80 per cent) of insured claim the benefit in cash and use it to buy private care, often from migrant individuals (European Commission 2018). Compared to Finland, the difference is remarkable. In Finland, a significant part of long-term care provision consists of public services, mainly home care services and serviced housing (Kestilä et al 2019, 199). In England, long-term care is means tested and therefore only those who cannot afford to buy the services they need from private markets are entitled to public care services or cash benefits. The social policies covering long-term care in these three respective countries result in very different outcomes for the citizens, for the workforce providing care, and for the state. In the case of long-term care, it could be argued that the social democratic welfare state acknowledges the ailment of all people in need of long-term care and carries the responsibility to provide for them. The German model also covers all citizens, but there is more emphasis on family, based on the subsidiarity idea whereby the responsibility is transferred to the lowest possible level of actors. Funding is based on income-related premiums, and the system offers flat-rate benefits in a given category of care needs (Nadash et al 2018). Ailment is thus recognised across social classes, but the family has a primary role in organising and paying for care, making the choice between family care and accessing the service more available for the better off. For the liberal model, in the case of long-term care, ailment is a public issue only when one cannot afford it by oneself. It would not be fair to portray liberal welfare states as always disregarding human ailment in their social policies. For example, the National Health Service (NHS) in England is a universal health service that covers all residents. Even if responding to ailment via public care provision is marginalised in the English social service sector, in the health service system, ailment is universally acknowledged. But even though different welfare state models or regimes help to analyse how ailment is regarded theoretically, the reality is always more complex.

Failing the ailing

During the relatively short period when the affluent welfare states expanded and strengthened social rights, the public and collective responses to ailment through social services and social policies in general were more extensive than ever before in the history of the modern world. After this period, social policies in many welfare states have undergone significant shifts that have been well documented by researchers studying transforming welfare states (for example Pierson 1994; Seeleib-Kaiser 2008; Ranci and Pavolini 2013). These shifts relate to changes in social policies, often due to austerity politics, and in changes in the organisation of care in the wider sociopolitical contexts of ailing.

In both Finland and the United Kingdom, these shifts are connected to the role of the public sector, which has undergone major reforms in both countries. A 'permanent austerity' (Pierson 2001) discourse now dominates the discussions about the public sector, its resources and its responsibilities. The focus in political discussions increasingly concerns the national economy and the economic competitiveness of the state (Wrede et al 2020). As Greener (2018, 2) argues, 'the main functions of social policy have become to alleviate the more extreme forms of poverty and to support corporations in the economy, with any claims that it should do more than this being dismissed as "unaffordable".' The well-being of the population is less in focus, and the essential role of the state is to ensure favourable circumstances for market actors. Parallel to the austerity discourse, a shift in social policies towards governance has fundamentally changed the role of the public actors in health and social care (see Newman and Clarke 2009). The emphasis on governance means that the role of the public sector has changed from a producer to a regulator of welfare state services (Jessop 1998). Simultaneously, the activation and integration of individuals, families, civil society, markets and the third sector has become a political and practical objective of social policies in multiple arenas, including education, health and social care, and employment policies (Newman and Tonkens 2011a). Janet Newman and Evelien Tonkens (2011a, 13–14) have described this shift as a 'new care and welfare order', its key pillars being choice, participation and responsibility. Collective responses to ailment have thus been formulated so that individuals seek the support and care they need from the markets that sell commodified (care) products.

There are various factors behind the changes in the role of the public sector and the welfare state, such as the ageing of the population, economic fluctuations and the rise of neoliberalism. The critique of the welfare state as a burden became common and loud as early as in 1950s' Britain. In the 1980s, the earlier aim of full employment was replaced by budget balancing, low inflation, a stable currency, and welfare state retrenchment, driven by Prime Minister Thatcher's administration (Hay 2004, 511). A central policy aim was to free markets from collective decision making and make employment relations more flexible. The welfare state was defined as being too expensive, bureaucratic, and creating welfare dependency instead of boosting self-reliance (Hemerjick 2012, 41). Since the 1990s, similar reforms in social and employment policies have been implemented in many European countries, not least due to the political influence of the European Union, which has reduced differences in national policies (for example Bernhard 2010; Hermann 2014).

If the 'golden age' of the welfare state was an era of decommodification, referring to the growing degree to which a person could maintain a livelihood without relying on the markets for welfare provision, the following period is characterised by re-commodification. This means that the well-being of individuals has again been made increasingly dependent on their labour market competitiveness – that is, their ability to sell their ability to work on the market. During the expansion period of the welfare state, the dependency on markets diminished. Public education and health services in the United Kingdom, and social services in the Nordic countries, targeted the entire population. During the regimes of Thatcher in the United Kingdom and Ronald Reagan in the United States, and after the recession of the 1990s in Finland, the tide turned. Public services were privatised, marketised and simply cut. Consequently, people and the public sector were ever more dependent on the market instead of on public services. An important strand of academic research has examined how drastically this shift towards markets eventually changed the core basis of the welfare state (for example Pierson 1994; Gilbert 2002; Powell and Hewitt 2002; Julkunen 2017). But despite the changes, there seems to be a consensus over a certain stability of the welfare state, a constant feature of which being the strong support that citizens still show for the welfare state in Nordic countries and in the United Kingdom (Julkunen 2017).

The popularity of the welfare state has not prevented the implementation of austerity policies, for example in Finland especially during and after the 1990s recession. These and other public sector reforms, such as marketisation, have been essential in making the care of older adults a key topic in social policy and economic policy debates. Of course, these debates have also been shaped by demographic transformations in the western world, that is, rapidly ageing populations. It took years of academic and political battle before care became a political issue and a target for policies – a social question that required a collective answer just as much as poverty does (Wilson 1977; Ungerson 1990; Orloff 1993; Anttonen and Zechner 2011). In the era of expansive welfare states, public resources were pooled for elder care. This also meant that during the economic downturn, or when political power relations changed, these resources could also be cut and redirected. After a short period of perceiving care as a social right, at least in the Nordic countries, it is increasingly being perceived as a burden in political discourses as well as in state budgets, and merely an economic cost for the public sector (for example Kröger 2019; Knickman and Snell 2002). Individual responsibility for one's ailment has replaced collective responsibility to some extent, and has been promoted via numerous free-choice, cash-for-care programmes, tax deductions, and similar arrangements throughout Europe (Meagher and Szebehely 2013; Ranci and Pavolini 2013).

These social policy instruments, such as service vouchers, individual budgets, and cash-for-care schemes, are promoted as granting more autonomy to service users. These have been introduced into care policies throughout Europe, including Finland and the United Kingdom (Ungerson and Yeandle 2007; Yeandle et al 2012). The empirical findings about the impact of free-choice models are neither uniform nor clear.

There is some evidence that having more freedom of choice does increase the recipient's sense of control, feeling of being empowered, and their satisfaction with services (for example Brown et al 2007; Glendinning et al 2008; Hatton and Waters 2011; Forder et al 2012; Harry et al 2017). Simultaneously, certain groups of people, such as older adults and the users of mental health services, do not self-evidently benefit from free choice (Glendinning et al 2008; Netten et al 2012; Eklund and Markström 2015). Since people seek care services when they depend on support and help, in these situations the need to exercise rational choice, find information and compare services can be a tall order. In situations of acute ailment, people practically need proxies such as family members who can make informed decisions on their behalf. For those who lack trustworthy and capable proxies, the benefits of free choice are not clear.

The instruments of free choice such as cash-for-care and voucher systems can also form liaisons with the markets and private enterprises, thus opening up possibilities for profit and marketing efforts, and the exploitation of 'customers' who can be in vulnerable positions. As market mechanisms, the instruments of free choice are also supported and promoted by international bodies such as the Organisation for Economic Co-operation and Development (OECD) (for example Lundsgaard 2005). Before the 1990s, the OECD hardly reported on care. But this started to change dramatically (see OECD 2022) as care increasingly became defined in policy and politics as an economic cost instead of as a social right. Large international private equity firms had barely anything to do with care in the 1980s, but now, many welfare states and their care systems are dependent on private care companies owned by multinational private equity firms (Meagher and Szebehely 2010; Burns et al 2016). Ailment is a global political issue, and in consequence of these changes in policy and politics, it has been subjugated to profit making and the transactions of global capital and venture, as we discuss in the next chapter.

In regard to the political and practical responses to ailment in social and care policies, ideas about humans as ailing beings have also changed to reflect the expectation of a greater responsibility and participation of individuals both in relation to themselves and to each other as members of their communities. These changes can be depicted through the idea of active citizenship. On the one hand, the strengthening of 'activity' discourses reflects transforming ideas concerning the relationship between individuals and the state (and other public authorities such as municipalities). This poses a question of who should be actively responding to human ailment. From this perspective, a shift from an active *state* to active *citizens* has taken place (Óskarsdóttir 2007, 27–8). On the other hand, the emphasis on 'activity' implies a shift from assumedly 'passive' citizens to 'active' ones (Johansson and Hvinden 2007, 33), reflecting the idea that previously the role of citizens was more passive, and that 'passive' citizens have now become targets of 'activation'. While contemporary states (and other public authorities) have to some extent withdrawn from concrete responses to human ailment, they have taken a new role in producing ever more active, responsible, independent and enterprising citizens through, for example, education (Siivonen and Brunila 2014; Brunila and Siivonen 2016) or labour market policies (Paju et al 2020). In particular, discourses that value 'active citizens' and stigmatise 'welfare dependency' are part of the broader neoliberal transformation and its criticism of the allegedly passivising welfare state (for example Wiggan 2012).

There is a striking resemblance to the punitive poorhouse system that we discussed earlier, whereby individuals depending on public support are defined as undeserving ailing individuals who may be punished and blamed for needing support and care – that is, they are punished and blamed for bothering (that is, ailing) others, including the economy. However, while a poorhouse was a concrete, materially visible and institutionally distinctive response to the ailments of the poor, the contemporary activation discourses are often more diffuse and hidden. Citizens are encouraged to become more active and self-responsible in various forums, including health services, various levels of education starting from kindergarten, therapy, free-time sports, self-help literature, news media, social media and so forth. Responses to human ailment are increasingly present in the everyday, and they are increasingly proactive and future oriented. While the poorhouse system was based on reacting to the acute ailments of the poor, the contemporary activation policies are increasingly based on the anticipation of various risks, and most importantly, the risk of ailment and dependency. Furthermore, the contemporary activation policies assume that active citizens need less collective care and support now, and more importantly, in the future. This ideal and expectation, however, ignores the fact that the care needs of ailing beings always tend to become actual in various moments of the life course, not least in advanced age.

What is perceived as 'activeness' depends of course on the underlying assumptions of what is seen as ideal by society. Certain relationships are considered more active than others, and in neoliberal discourses, for example, being a customer or a consumer in markets is seen as being more active than being a patient or client of a public service. But what might seem a more active approach at the policy level may look very different in the everyday lives of individuals with ailments. For example, in the Nordic home care services, there used to be a lot of flexibility in the home care encounter, which meant that the home care worker and the person needing care were able to define the content of the home care services through the actual encounter, making choices and participating in their own care (Szebehely 2003; Vabø and Szebehely 2012). In the 2020s, as home care services are organised according to market principles, activity is often understood as acts by a consumer who makes choices in the care market, for example by choosing care products and providers.

Paradoxically, in the actual home care encounter, this means more rigid practices, and therefore a more passive role for the person in need of care as they are not allowed to influence the care that they need according to situated needs, but have to rely on purchasing relatively fixed care products from the market (Vamstad 2016; Ward et al 2020). Difficulties in exercising choice are part and parcel of the retrenchment of the welfare state and cutbacks in funding and services. These have contributed to increasingly unequal access to health and social care, as those with greater financial resources have better access to services, and those who lack financial resources more frequently do not have their social and health care needs met (Van Aerschot 2014; Manderbacka et al 2018; Kröger et al 2019). Again, as in Ancient Greece, the ailment of the elites seems to deserve more attention than the ailment of other social classes.

It is good, however, to keep in mind that in all societies, personal and familial responsibility is the predominant source of support for individuals who face ailments. Another persistent trend is the increasing construction of 'older adults' as a specific subject, and increasingly as a target of public policy. Regarding older persons, the overall trend seems to be from the gradual acknowledgement of individual needs and rights during the era of expansive welfare states, to the contemporary mixtures of demographic alarmism, personal responsibilisation, and the politics of free choice. Responsibilisation in this context means that at least some of the public responsibility for providing, arranging, funding and the oversight of the quality of care has been shifted to individuals. Regarding the governance of ailment, the governance of old age is thus a key question in contemporary, ageing societies.

To conclude this chapter, one could say that while the ways in which ailment is governed vary in time and place, an overall trend in the developed welfare states is a continuum that begins from sanctions and very basic maintenance; and progresses to a more public provision and then to market commodity and personal responsibility. Through the history of social and care policy, the idea that ailment is a human trait worthy of collective attention and action has become stronger. However, responding to ailment has also been subordinate to other interests, such as governing the workforce and enhancing economic productivity. Next, we will further explore what happens when human ailment becomes governed through marketisation and markets.

THREE

Profit making and ailment: the marketisation and financialisation of care

At the time of writing, in 2021, it is not exactly front-page news that an overall economic shift has taken place in care policies in many western countries, where the heyday of the welfare state is long gone. This shift and its effects have been conceptualised and reviewed as the marketisation of care (Anttonen and Häikiö 2011; Meagher and Szebehely 2013). Marketisation means the implementation of market logic and practices in public care services (Anttonen and Meagher 2013). As we discuss in this chapter, this may take various forms. It has also been established that while marketisation is a significant part of the economic shift, the change consists of multiple ongoing processes in how care is organised. We argue that these processes significantly affect the politics of ailment by replacing the ailing subject with an active market actor as the target of social policies (Hoppania et al 2016), and by changing the ways profits are made in the field of care (Hoppania et al 2022). As discussed in the previous chapter, the ways in which social policies that emphasise marketisation recognise, rationalise and govern human ailment dramatically differ from the social policies of the expanding welfare state. Nevertheless, ailment continues to be a mobilising force that simultaneously generates both social and care relations and market and financial activity.

In this chapter we examine how marketisation and, as we later argue, increasingly the financialisation of care transform the social orders which emerged as collective and public answers to ailment during the golden era of the welfare state (see previous chapter). Following Krippner's (2005, 174) definition, we define financialisation as 'a pattern of accumulation in which profits accrue primarily through financial channels', rather than through service or commodity production.

Marketisation and financialisation are replacing the idea of collective responsibility for care by introducing the mechanisms of profit making, competition and choice as solutions to human ailment. These processes are based on politics that assume and expect people to embrace a figure of the human-being as an entrepreneurial and self-investing subject, instead of an ailing individual (see also Hoppania and Vaittinen 2015). In these processes and politics, ailments are mere temporary hiccups to be dealt with through self-preparation and the purchase of care services and products such as insurance. If the prospect of getting old and needing care troubles and bothers people, this ailing is handled by market solutions. Individuals are urged to invest in insurance, supportive social ties and their own health, so that if care needs emerge at an older age, they can be handled individually by relying on family members and markets, instead of the welfare state (see also Newman and Tonkens 2011b, 180–1). At the same time, austerity politics have moved resources away from the public actors that provide social care, giving market actors opportunities to tap into ailment as a source of profit.

The problem with these policy trends and the neoliberal vision on which they rely is that the logic of the market is different from, and is largely incompatible with, those responses to ailment which are based on the logic of care (Mol 2008). Markets and market actors stress self-interest, profit making and competition, whereas care is based on (at times altruistic) concern for the well-being of others. Markets also require delineated products to buy and sell, whereas ailment and the logic of care are about interdependency, relationality, and changing needs and situations (Hoppania et al 2021). When care for ailing bodies and people in need of care is brought into the sphere of markets and finance, ailment as a core part of human life is commodified and subjugated to profit making. While businesses perceive ailment as producing unlimited market opportunities, they fail in the more profound recognition of ailment as an existential human condition warranting ethically sound responses such as affordable care.

The field of care policies is going through various parallel transitions of marketisation and financialisation, and the concomitant processes of commodification, privatisation and responsibilisation (Brennan et al 2012; Burns et al 2016; Anttonen and Karsio 2017; Vaittinen et al 2018). Marketisation and the financialisation of care fade out ailment as basis for social rights, making it also difficult to politically steer care provision governed by market logic. Paradoxically, ailment simultaneously activates the interests of for-profit companies that participate in finding solutions for increasing care needs. This is the new social order that marketisation and the financialisation of care are creating. To understand this argument, we discuss what the marketisation and financialisation of care mean, and explore these developments through the lens of ailment.

Marketisation of care

Marketisation of care is part of the overall marketisation of society and government that began as early as the 1970s in liberal welfare states such as Australia and the United Kingdom, and expanded to other welfare states including the Nordic countries in the 1980s and 1990s (Clarke 2006; Meagher and Szebehely 2013; Fine and Davidson 2018). Here, we use the notion of the marketisation of care as an umbrella term that entails the political and practical changes and transitions that transform care services, practices and structures into market goods and products. Marketisation typically includes private service provision: for-profit companies provide publicly funded services through outsourcing and competitive bidding processes (Anttonen and Meagher 2013). However, market-based practices may also be utilised within the public sector, without (or before) outsourcing services. Marketisation may mean that market rationalities and practices are brought inside the public sector care provision, especially by implementing management practices such as increased competition between care units, standardised work processes, hierarchical planning, and formalised surveillance and control systems of care workers, originally developed for factory work management (Hoppania et al 2021).

Public and non-profit care providers and users of care services are assumed to act as if embedded in a market context governed by economic logic. These transitions refer to transforming public administration into something mimicking business administration, increasing public service production by for-profit actors, and changing the role of the service user towards primarily a consumer, instead of a citizen with welfare rights (Clarke et al 2007; Anttonen and Häikiö 2011; Brennan et al 2012; Anttonen and Meagher 2013; Vaittinen et al 2018). The transition from public to private is not a one-dimensional change from public to market provision (Walker 1984), and instead, marketisation takes varying forms (Gingrich 2011). Marketisation results in different types of care systems, in which the power relations and responsibilities between the state (or municipality/local council), the private producer, and the service user vary. However, one thing is common to all these varieties of publicly governed marketised care: that care becomes commodified and the idea of an ailing individual is replaced by an idea(l) of a rational and self-serving *homo economicus*.

Through markets, care 'becomes more a commodity than a relationship' (Fine and Davidson 2018, 512). Care is thus a commodity sold and bought in the markets that exist in order to create economic surplus (Dahl 2017). Consequently, marketisation will 'ultimately change society's conception of care' (Fine and Davidson 2018, 512). These concerns are similar to ours. As collective responses to ailment become dependent on competition and choice rather than the equal treatment of ailing individuals, ailment is slowly subjugated to market interest. Earlier we defined marketisation as all the practices and policies which turn care into a market good or commodity. If we take a closer look at these transitions on the national level historically, and take England and Finland as the main examples, a more detailed understanding of marketisation emerges. The marketisation of care, and more generally social and health services, has mainly consisted of two waves: first, the outsourcing of public services to private producers; and second, increasing user choice and cash-for-care schemes in publicly funded, or at least subsidised, services (Anttonen and Karsio 2017).

In examining the marketisation of Finnish and English elder care systems, we must take into consideration that the English system is means tested or income tested, whereas the Finnish system is universal so that the entry to services is needs tested (Morgan and Zechner 2022). This difference has implications for analysing these systems and their marketisation. That is, the starting point for marketisation to take place, as well as the ways in which ailment is societally perceived and recognised, is different in the respective countries. While in England roughly half of the older adults in care homes are fully self-funded (Jarret 2019b), in Finland the share is close to 0 per cent; hence these countries represent very different systems. On the other hand, and somewhat paradoxically in the context of the universal ideals, the Finnish public system for elder care may include extremely high user fees based on the older adult's income. For example, in publicly funded long-term residential care facilities, the residents' fees are up to 85 per cent of their monthly income (Act on Social and Health Care

User Fees 734/1992). Even if the services are not means tested, but needs tested, the final costs for the Finnish care user and English care user might be the same. The main difference is that if a person fails the financial assessment in England, they will not receive public services and are on their own, whereas in Finland everybody passing the needs assessment is entitled to a public service. Therefore, in Finland, responding to the ailment of older people is perceived as a public responsibility and receiving care a universal right, in contrast to the English care model. Both countries also offer support for covering the costs of care either through funding support (England) or by lowering the user fees (Finland) for those passing the care needs assessment. An essential difference is that in England service users may need to sell their housing to cover the user fees, whereas in Finland the Act on Social and Health Care Fees (734/1992) does not require this.

In England, housing assets may be needed, particularly by self-funders. The Competition and Markets Authority (CMA) published a report revealing that self-funding care home customers in England paid 41 per cent higher fees compared to customers funded by the local authority (Jarrett 2019a, 22). This raises another question about the economic and financial status of for-profit providers, of whether they are funding publicly subsidised customers by charging higher fees to the self-funders? This is called cross-subsidisation (Jarrett 2019a, 22) and it further enables profit making from individual ailment. Until recently, this has been difficult to investigate, since while prices paid by local authorities (for those users who qualify for state support) are available, the prices that self-funders pay for their care home places have been unavailable (Allan et al 2021). This lack of transparency is one of the consequences of marketisation, as companies can appeal to protect business secrets, which allows them to covertly extract higher revenues from self-funded clients. Appealing to business secrecy also hinders the oversight and control that the state or local council (municipalities in Nordic countries) are supposed to practise – after all, private care providers are also producing public goods and using public funds in that cause.

Cash-for-care systems, personal budgets, and the overall personalisation of care are a perfect avenue and arena to marketise and commodify care and ailment. Public social care budgets have been reduced substantially, and people are encouraged to pursue more individualised approaches and solutions (Morgan and Zechner 2022). The system of a personal budget offers the customer a budget to use for purchasing purposeful aid and services. The budget can be given to customers who can then use the money in the way they want, or it can be managed by a case manager, who, together with the customer, makes decisions about the aid and services that are needed. However, in England at least, scant personal budgets leave the responsibility for organising, paying and the oversight of care to the individuals and their relatives (Bottery and Babalola 2020). Additionally, when previous care arrangements are portrayed as old-fashioned and stiff, they can be closed down without providing new services of the same coverage, as Caroline Needham (2014) has shown in relation to day centres for older adults.

These examples demonstrate how the public governing of ailment has shifted the focus from supporting individuals and families to meet the needs of care (by offering services) towards advising them to spend money wisely in care markets (Zechner 2017). The commodified services sold and bought in the market are then a site for companies to make profit from ailment. Moreover, individuals bear the responsibility of their choices, including their bad choices (Rostgaard 2006), which increases the risks related to care. This is unsatisfactory since care needs are difficult to foresee and they tend to change by the day. Thus, a care product bought one day may not be suitable the next. The logic of the market does not recognise this since what has already been purchased is not easily changeable. As the need for care increases as care service users ail over time, the cost for care incrementally increases, while income in older age rarely does. The slicing-up of commodified care products creates almost unlimited business opportunities at the individual's expense, and in the worst cases this can lead to personal bankruptcy and a severe lack of sufficient care.

In addition to responsibility for oversight, responsibility for funding may also be shifted to individuals, for example by requiring citizens to buy care insurance (see Newman and Tonkens 2011b, 180–1). Finland is witnessing an ideological shift in that both economic research institutes and non-governmental organisations have begun to campaign for individual preparation for old age through financial means and healthy lifestyles (VTKL 2019). ETLA – an economic research institute funded by the largest Finnish employers' association – promotes freedom of choice in long-term care in old age by long-term care insurance and by part-release of housing equity (ETLA 2020). Neoliberal economics often perceives public responses to ailment as a costly burden, and the responsibility to prepare for unforeseen misfortune is shifted to individuals. In this thinking, the market is created as an answer to individuals for preparing against, for example, illness, unemployment and old age. Hence, ailment as a productive force is at work here. The neoliberal political answers to bothering and ailing relations generate markets where new hierarchies around ailment emerge. In these markets, ailment may also be economically exploited – benefiting some, but leaving many people and aspects of ailment neglected.

Ailment often results in care policies that combine market and public resources. Examples from long-term care insurance systems from Japan and Germany illustrate the productive power of ailment. Japan chose to introduce a mandatory public long-term care insurance (LTCI) in 2000. The ageing of the population, the erosion of the traditional family due to fewer children per household, more women in employment, and the gradual changing of norms prompted the implementation of long-term care insurance (Campbell et al 2010). This insurance is financed by a combination of social insurance premiums, paid by all persons aged 40 and over according to income, and taxes. The main goal was to support older adults in living a dignified and independent life. Additionally, market-related objectives were present, such as allowing for-profit companies to enter the previously bureaucratic system, in order to increase competition and consumer choice. Another motivation was to create savings in medical spending, since before the long-term care insurance was implemented, large numbers of older adults resided in hospitals (Tamiya et al 2011).

Marketisation has also been one motivation behind the German public long-term care insurance since 1995 (Theobald 2012). Previously, non-profit welfare associations were the main service providers, but the long-term care insurance paved the way for market-based for-profit service providers. An alarming consequence was that the advocacy function of welfare associations weakened, since it was separated from service provision. The working conditions of care workers became worse after the insurance was introduced, it became more difficult to attract voluntary workers, and voluntary work became increasingly monetarised (Theobald 2012). In Germany, the public insurance may also be supplemented with additional voluntary private insurance, and the contributions are subsidised by the government (Gori and Morciano 2019). This means that there can be different tiers of beneficiaries, with some receiving better compensation levels than others. The tax-funded social assistance system pays for the uncovered costs of care services for individuals lacking sufficient funds. Half of all beneficiaries choose cash benefits instead of services (Gori and Morciano 2019). Persons electing for cash receive less than half the value of the service benefits, but the use of cash is unrestricted (Cuellar and Wiener 2000). Care work as a response to ailment is thus still predominantly managed by families in Germany.

Long-term care insurance may have changed care arrangements more dramatically in Japan than in Germany. The public system of social care for older adults was meagre before the long-term care insurance, and the emphasis on care by family members has been historically strong in Japan. The oldest son, and in practice the wife of the oldest son, have been the main people responsible for taking care of older family members. The traditional Japanese societal response to ailment is thus based on social relations and cultural norms. The norm has been very strong, and failure to comply may have resulted in feelings of guilt and sanctions from the members of kin or other social networks (Schultz Lee 2010). Hence it may have been assumed by policy makers that the long-term care insurance would not necessarily have increased the demand for services. Care as a response to the ailment of older adults was seen as a family issue, although medical coverage was still good. However, the demand for services has increased exponentially since the introduction of long-term care insurance (Tamiya et al 2011; Ikegami 2019).

Japan's example demonstrates how collective solutions for ailment are needed. Such insurances with premiums to pay, and as in Germany the opportunity to supplement the public insurance with a private one, also function as reminders for individuals about the costs of care and provide incentives for individual preparation for ailments, hence privatising responsibility (Ha et al 2017). They thus tap into ailment by monetising the feelings of dread and trouble that people have about their ageing selves and relatives. Indeed, the private long-term care insurance market is seen as a very attractive market for investors; for example, in the United States, there is little regulation, and expenditure levels are about 150 billion dollars per year (Kaye 2009; Huang et al 2021). Also, 28 per cent of community care and as many as 75 per cent of nursing home service users pay out of pocket (Kaye et al 2009, 17). For an individual, annual out-of-pocket expenditure for nursing home care can easily be over 70,000 dollars (Huang et al 2021), and one in ten will incur out-of-pocket long-term care expenses in excess of 200,000 dollars (Braun et al 2019). Thus, when ailing is mainly addressed in the markets, this can generate profits for insurance companies, although the market in the United States is in decline. In 2000 there were 125 insurance companies selling private long-term care insurance, whereas in 2019 only 15 were left (Moench and Stender 2020). Only about 10 per cent of those aged 62 and over have private long-term care insurance and the insurance now has a low level of take-up at all wealth levels. While lower-income groups cover their long-term care expenses with public Medicaid, the better off refrain from buying long-term care insurance due to high administrative costs and adverse selection (Braun et al 2019).

Another step in marketisation is the domination of large for-profit nursing home chains in long-term care provision. Large for-profit nursing homes are characterised by property being separated from other operations, activities that are globally dispersed in many locations, and companies often being based in tax havens, as we expand on in the next section. A comparison of for-profit nursing home chains in Canada, Norway, Sweden, the United Kingdom and the United States demonstrates that large for-profit nursing home chains are often owned by private equity investors, have undergone many ownership changes over time, and possess complicated organisational structures (Harrington et al 2017). The nursing home chains tend to have large revenues with high profit margins, and governments and the public find it difficult to obtain information on their ownership, costs and quality of services (Harrington et al 2017). The oversight and control over quality has become more fragmented than before and rests largely on the shoulders of individuals. Evidence from Sweden indicates that professionals who bring up problems with services tend to be met with silence from supervisors and directors. Furthermore, taking the issue to a higher level for investigation results in stigmatisation and often has severe consequences for the careers of those who bring the issues up (Hedin and Månsson 2012). This is, therefore, yet another example of how for-profit companies move away from responding to ailment with care as the core of their policies.

So far we have discussed various examples of the marketisation of care as a response to ailment in neoliberal times. This has created new social orders emerging around care. These market-friendly responses are a basis for publicly funded care markets where for-profit companies provide care as a market commodity for public sector actors, such as municipalities and local councils, as well as for citizens. Marketisation policies enable private providers to make profit from individual and collective ailment. Ultimately, the figure of the ailing subject as a bearer of social rights is replaced with an idea of a non-ailing, active citizen-consumer (cf Clarke et al 2007). Disturbingly, this self-feeding process of turning human ailment into a sellable and buyable commodity is not limited to national care policies, but is expanding into global financial markets, as we shall discuss in the next section.

Financialisation of care

The financialisation of care refers to processes through which care becomes an avenue for profit making by financial means. In particular, financialised care has little to do with actual care provision and care work. The marketisation of care points to the introduction of competition, market practices, and market logic into the organisation and production of public services, whereas the notion of financialised care draws attention to actors who are motivated by financial ends (for example care companies owned by venture capitalists) and who utilise financial tools (for example inter-company loans, tax avoidance) in their operational logic, while integrating these frequently hidden actions in the production of public care services (Hoppania et al 2022). Even though marketisation and financialisation of care are two separate processes, there are many overlaps between them, and in practice financialisation implies marketisation.

Natascha van der Zwan (2014) offers an analytical framework for the study of financialisation by differentiating its three aspects, reflecting how it is used in financialisation literature. First, the 'emergence of a new regime of accumulation' refers to the emergence of growing financial activities of and within for-profit care companies. Second, 'the ascendancy of the shareholder value orientation' points to the relations and processes within corporations (van der Zwan 2014, 102, 107–10). It also means foregrounding corporate interest in shareholder value over the value of other *stakeholders*, such as workers, managers, public entities purchasing services, clients and their families (Hoppania et al 2022). Third, 'the financialisation of everyday life' concerns processes whereby the citizen emerges as an investor in policy discourses and practices, as financial products penetrate the daily lives of the population through private pension plans, reverse mortgages, and consumer credit (cf van der Zwan 2014, 111–14).

Financialisation of care is preceded by the growth of private care markets. Without private for-profit care provision, there are no opportunities for finances to take over. The 'emergence of a new regime of accumulation' is therefore based on the marketisation of care. The existence of a growing care market is obvious even at a glance at the statistics of care provision. In England, the new regime evolved earlier than in the Nordic welfare states. According to Tim Jarrett (2019b), in 1984, 57 per cent of places in the English residential care sector were in care homes run by local authorities; 26 per cent were provided by the private sector; and 17 per cent were in the voluntary sector. In 2017, just 8 per cent of places were in local authority-run care homes; 76 per cent were in the private sector; and 17 per cent were in the voluntary sector. Thus, from 1984 to 2017 the care sector in England transformed almost completely from public to private production.

The emergence of the private care market took place later in Finland. In 1990 the private for-profit care market was practically non-existent, with 88 per cent of all social services – which includes elder care – being provided by the public sector; 12 per cent by the non-profit private sector; and less than

1 per cent by the for-profit private sector (Karsio and Anttonen 2013). In 2018 the public sector provided 64 per cent; the non-profit private sector 16 per cent; and the for-profit private sector 20 per cent of all social services. But in residential care, the share of private producers was more significant, with 34 per cent being provided by for-profit companies and 19 per cent by non-profits (data compiled by the authors from Tevameri 2020; 2021).

The examples from England and Finland demonstrate that as publicly provided care is marketised and outsourced to private for-profit companies according to the neoliberal care policies, a new market is created. The mostly publicly funded care market thus provides new opportunities for companies that previously had no profit-making opportunities in the field of care. The bigger the market is, the bigger the players are. Consequently, the larger multinational companies owned by private equity firms are more capable of and willing to use financial means to make profit, as we will argue next.

In focusing on financialisation in the context of marketisation, it is crucial to see that profits related to ailment and care provision accrue increasingly through global financial channels, rather than through regular trade in commodities or services. The growing financial activities of non-financial firms and the increasing significance of finance in the economy must therefore be scrutinised (van der Zwan 2014, 103–6). Financial activities mean that profits are not gained so much from production, or even from investing in the production of goods or services, but from interest, dividends and capital gains, which are becoming larger and more common. Not only is there a new or bigger market; the structure of the private market is also changing. The concentration of the market in a few large international private equity-owned for-profit consolidated companies is a prime example of both the emergence of a new regime of accumulation, and also the ascendancy of shareholder value orientation. In the Nordic countries, especially in Sweden and to some extent in Finland, a few large companies have sought, and continue to seek, to increase their market share (Erlandsson et al 2013; Karsio and Anttonen 2013; Harrington et al 2017; Tevameri 2020; Hoppania et al 2022).

As Diane Burns and others (2016) have demonstrated, the trend is similar in England, even though care homes have historically been small-scale businesses. Larger companies have the financial means to generate profits not only by selling care services, but also by utilising the complex structures of multinational firms and internal debt arrangements to make profits and exercise tax avoidance. Internal debt arrangements and the tax avoidance of multinational firms in the context of care and ailment work at a distance from the ailing body of an older person in need of care. Despite this, a new regime of accumulation of profit has emerged, stemming from human ailment. A multinational, multibillion private equity firm is not responsible for the care of a single individual, neither is it bothered by the ailing bodies of older adults. Nevertheless, national care systems are becoming increasingly dependent on the actions of such companies. Since closing down care homes would risk the lives of their inhabitants, states subsequently become hostages to such companies (Hudson 2014).

As private equity enters the market of care, so does the prominence and promotion of shareholder value as a guiding principle of corporate behaviour (van der Zwan 2014, 107–10) in care services. This aspect of financialisation focuses on the redistribution processes within corporations, that is, between managers, shareholders and employees. It means that the operation of care homes becomes a new arena in which to develop corporate efficiency, and the key goal is to maximise dividends and keep stock prices high. In the care sector, this has led to processes which sometimes have grave consequences for workers and the service users. Workloads have been intensified in order to meet performance and productivity targets, and the productivity increases have often been used for the benefit of the corporation or the shareholders rather than being fed into wages (Cushen and Thompson 2016). As Amy Horton

(2022, 154) has discussed, financialised elder care provision systematically relies on labour to absorb financialised pressure, however, 'care's labour intensity deters the continued expansion of companies even where financing is available'. In practice this means that when shareholder value is sought from cuts in labour costs, problems in care quality are bound to emerge. Moreover, in a labour-intensive field such as care services, decreasing the number of staff is an easy way of cutting costs, while increasing short-term profits. Saving on salaries contributes to the 'trimming' of these financialised care companies into a condition where the companies themselves are 'fit' to be sold to the next capital investor. When combined with complex tax planning and debt leverages, these mechanisms increase the profits of the shareholders more efficiently than the profits gained solely through the production of services (Hoppania et al 2022).

The ascendancy of the shareholder value orientation can be interpreted in different ways in the context of ailment. If marketisation transforms care and care work into sellable and buyable products to provide an opportunity to make profit by buying and selling the product, the shareholder value effect instead focuses on making profit by increasing the value of the shares by whatever means possible. All activities are thus planned to increase shareholder value, rather than producing high-quality care services. As Joseph Vogl (2017, 160) argues about financial markets, 'systematic risk is transferred downwards'. Firstly, this means in practice that whereas the public sector as the purchaser of care services, or a citizen buying services out of pocket, expects that the contract between the service provider and purchaser guides the relationship between the care service user and the service provider, in reality, shareholder value steers and directs the private provider's actions. The shareholder's risk is limited to losing the value of the shares, whereas the public body carries the risk of not providing care to ailing citizens, and individuals carry the risk of making sound choices to receive proper care.

Secondly, as citizens, taxpayers, service users themselves, and their relatives can be actual shareholders of care companies, they might end up in a dual role. A person receiving care in an outsourced publicly funded service might be at the same time a service user, paying for the service through tax and/ or user fees, and additionally a shareholder in the private company producing the service. Furthermore, the person can also be an investor and shareholder in the company that owns the facilities and rents them to the private service provider. Thus, these two imaginary service users may be in an unequal position in relation to each other, if one is a shareholder and the other is not. This dual role connects to the financialisation of everyday life: that is, seeing and identifying citizens as investors and financial actors even when they are ailing, in the context of potential or actual need for care. The emphasis in the financialisation of care is on individual responsibility and calculative assessment in financial management. But in the context of ailment, the role of an ailing citizen entitled to care is transformed into one of a rational and capable market and financial actor.

Ailment in its meaning of 'troubling' or 'bothering' also applies here. Ailment's affective dimensions demonstrate how ailment bothers people. Yet the fact that everybody is ailing and can at any moment fall ill is being financialised. If the public promise of care is vague, it cannot be trusted. Private insurance is sold for a range of health-related conditions, and increasingly there are discussions about how individuals could and should prepare for ageing. Thus, citizens are defined as investors (van der Zwan 2014, 111–13), and their troubling fears regarding their future are used for profit making and thus turned into capital. Here, the systematic risks are again transferred downwards. While officially, at least in Nordic countries, the public promise to care for the citizens when they are no longer able to care for themselves is strong, the reality is laden with scandalously bad care services (Lloyd et al 2014; Jönson 2016; Hjelt 2019). For example, various private care homes and major care companies were involved in a care scandal in Finland in 2019, and news broke that numerous privately owned care homes had been placed under public inspection for several years, but improvements were not made. After the scandal became public, more serious problems in other private care homes were detected: systematic understaffing; and including retired workers, deceased people and even cartoons as 'ghost' workers in rosters (Hjelt 2019). The scandal affected one of the largest care companies so drastically that it was acquired by its creditors. Markedly, care scandals are in stark contrast with the Nordic universalist ideal of care that is attractive, affordable and available to all social classes (Vabø and Szebehely 2012).

If the Nordic countries are only now facing care scandals deriving from marketisation and financialisation, England is already established as a prime example of what marketisation and financialisation of care can result in. The entire field of social care is currently in crisis, and more than anything, it is a funding and provision crisis. The private for-profit companies have not been able to produce quality care with the public funding allocated to them and at the same time make profits. Consequently, the public administration in charge of arranging care has faced the problem presented by marketisation critics from the beginning of this trend, of what to do when the for-profit companies face insolvency, which ought normally to be anticipated in markets. Since insolvencies of care homes would cause a humanitarian crisis if they were closed abruptly, the English public sector has thus far reacted by increasing their funding (Burns et al 2016; Glasby et al 2020).

To conclude, the financialisation of care and ailment is fundamentally changing the dynamics and interrelationships between market actors, the public sector, and individuals. In financialisation terms, as the new regime of accumulation expands, more financially motivated actors enter the field of care. Consequently, the publicly funded care services and individuals seeking care become more dependent on the private market, and thus on the large private equity-owned care companies; companies, whose motives are based on increasing shareholder value and making profit by financial means. Simultaneously, the financialisation of everyday life and ailment is changing the discourse, even in Nordic welfare states; An entrepreneurial, investing subject is created and the role of personal responsibility in responding to care needs is emphasized. This is part of a neoliberal project, which aims to create and strengthen individuals as subjects who respond to economic incentives in a predictable manner (Madra and Adaman 2013). Here, not only is the risk of ever-present ailment individualised, but the individual risk needs to be addressed by economic means, by saving and investing, and ultimately generating profits from the ailment of others or oneself.

Profiting from ailment

The concept of ailment opens the viewpoint of one's whole life as fundamentally ailing. In this sense, it raises somewhat contradictory points. Ailment cannot be contained in markets or via financial products since it is an existential, bodily, affective and relational fact of life that should be recognised and accepted as such. By examining the changes in care through the analytical framework of financialisation and marketisation in the context of ailment, we have demonstrated the drastic transformation of care from a public common good to a financialised market commodity. Ailment has largely been shunted from the locality of welfare states into the global flows of assets. Financialisation and the marketisation of care dramatically change the rationalities that justify the collective responses to ailment. If ailing bodies are to become objects of global financial activities and motives, the national care systems are in danger of losing their original purpose: collectively taking care of ailing individuals.

Making profit from human ailment is not a totally new phenomenon. Paid nurses, maids and babysitters have historically been part of the everyday life of the upper classes. Nevertheless, these arrangements have not been based on making profit for private companies or increasing shareholder value, but rather on providing a livelihood for individuals. In welfare states with extensive public care systems, providing collective answers with a reliance on multinational financialised firms is something the field of care has not witnessed before. The relationality of ailment emerges in these new neoliberal arrangements creating social orders around care, resulting in new divisions of risk and responsibility. Ailment, thus, not only creates collective and private responses for ailing individuals in the form of care, but it stirs up financial and market activities, which follow entirely different logic from the logic of care.

The neoliberal and financially driven approach to ailment differs from the universalist ideas of the Nordic welfare states, which have taken on the overall responsibility for ailment by offering a wide range of services and other kinds of support for those older adults in need of care (Vabø and Szebehely 2012). The transformation of ailment into a market commodity to be sold and bought by allegedly free and rational actors (that is, *homo economicus*) contributes to the de-politicisation of ailment as a private and seemingly (but falsely) non-ideological business issue. This erodes the idea of ailment as a public and explicitly political issue governed through deliberate decision making and democratic institutions. The financialisation of ailment further means that the entirety of the human being, the ailing body and mind, are subsumed in the global flows of finance, and individuals are expected to be or to become financially wise and make wise choices according to the logic of the market (for example Price and Livsey 2013). In the traditional universal welfare state model, the citizen is expected to contribute through work and paying taxes, and then they can expect that their care needs in old age will be met by society at least to a certain extent. This means that the need to rely on family or the market would be minimal: in other words, care is decommodified (Bambra 2005). The neoliberal model of the financialisation of care means that ailment and generalised care needs are privatised, that they rest on the individual, and that they are to a great extent handled in the market through economic transactions. By this process, care is thus recommodified (Leira and Saraceno 2006).

The care policies of recent decades have shifted so that the ageing and ailing citizenry is seen to trouble and ail the state in a way that endangers state economies. The public response has been to shift the responsibility of care increasingly onto individuals by means of marketisation and financialisation. Therein lies a conflict as ailing bodies and generalised care needs create new business opportunities and markets for financial and market actors, but are nevertheless still seen as a burden on the national economy. At the same time, this change has served to change the discourse of ailment and care so that ailment becomes increasingly more stigmatised. Not only is it undesirable to have various ailments, but if an individual has not prepared for and organised the care of such possible ailments, it is their own fault if they end up in need and requiring care that is not available or is out of reach because they cannot afford it. This approach increases inequalities since differences in income, health, assets, skills and education affect how people can prepare for ailment (see also Timonen 2016). But the inequalities deriving from marketisation and financialisation concern not only the ailing individuals in need of care, but also the caregivers, as we will demonstrate in the next chapter.

FOUR

Ailment in caring encounters and divisions of care labour

In the previous chapters we have examined human ailment as a force that throughout history has mobilised individuals, communities, public policies, and markets to respond. This chapter focuses on care relations and demonstrates how ailment mobilises concrete, embodied and emotional responses in immediate social encounters, along with gendered, racialised and classed divisions of labour that extend to the global scale. Throughout this book we have argued that as ailing subjects, human beings are always productive in ways that exceed productivity as it is commonly understood as a clear and measurable, economic relationship between an input and an output. Ailment of course has effects, but these effects are not usually isolated products or entities. Rather, they are relationships between actors, including those between caregivers and care receivers, or citizens and the state. The same relationality also applies to care, as a specific response to ailment. As Susan Himmelweit (2007, 583) argues, care 'has specific features that distinguish it from the economic activities involved in the provision of many other goods and services'. Intrinsic in care is the developed relationship, 'not the production of an output that is separable from the person delivering it' (Himmelweit 2007, 583). In emphasising the significance of relationality, our thinking thus builds on existing theories of care (for example Fisher and Tronto 1990; Kittay 2005).

The innumerable, varying responses to ailment in the world may be imagined as an emergent and constantly changing network of relatedness that organises societies (see also Dahl 2017). Moreover, responses to ailment are never entirely repetitive, or entirely similar to earlier responses. The ailments that individuals encounter are always particular and therefore call for different kinds of response. Care needs, especially, are always somewhat unpredictable, individual and mutable, because mental and bodily ailment appears differently in different people, and vary in different situations and at different points in time, even in the same person (Wærness 1984; Fisher and Tronto 1990; Mol 2008). It is also never certain how a body will respond to care, so the relations through which ailment is responded to are also particular and constantly changing. The way an individual responds to another person's ailment today will have consequences for their relationship tomorrow, albeit not entirely predictable consequences. There is thus considerable variety in human responses to ailment, and a large degree of unpredictability in the chains of reaction that ailment, as a mobilising force, creates. Through their various responses to ailment, including care, neglect, violence and humiliation, humans also actualise – or fail to actualise – their capacity to act and simultaneously constitute their moral, ethical and political identities. None of this, however, takes place in a social vacuum and only between individuals. The responses that ailment mobilises are always channelled through institutions, policies and societal structures.

In this chapter we first examine how ailment mobilises affective and embodied responses in concrete and immediate encounters of long-term care, between those who are ailing and need care, and those who respond to this ailment by providing care. Ailment refers to the bothering that troubles, afflicts and plagues the body and its embodied mind. Ailment, thus, has an affective dimension. We analyse this dimension from the starting point that ailment, as an unpredictable and changing force, brings up all kinds of responses – including new ailments. We refer to these new ailments as *caregiver ailment* in the vein of Main's (1957, 140) *staff ailment*, by which he means 'the distress suffered by patients' attendants'. With this concept we continue the work of ethicists of care who have called attention to caregivers as deserving of care, such as respite and the fulfilment of their own needs, which often remain unmet while caring for others (for example Kittay 2005, 459–60). Kittay has pointed out that conflict between the needs of care receivers and caregivers – both being oppressed groups – is an ethical dilemma that persists as long as societies are built on the perception that ailments and care needs are the exception to the norm of independence (cf Kittay 2005, 467). By focusing on ailment, we aim to overcome the separation or conflict between those in need of care and those providing it. Instead, we conceive of both as ailing beings with complex affective capacities.

The notion of affects emphasises the immanent social nature of emotions as an alternative to a merely psychological understanding of emotions (for example Massumi 1995; Clough 2008; Reckwitz 2012). Affects refer to 'those processes of life and vitality which circulate and pass between bodies' (Blackman 2012, 26), and affection to the bodily capacity to affect and be affected through impressions on our bodies caused by external bodies (not only human), as originally proposed by Spinoza in *Ethics* (1677/1982).

Like ailment, affect is thus intrinsically part of the relations between bodies, whether individual or collective (see Sointu 2016; Kolehmainen and Juvonen 2018, 3). Affect is located neither completely inside nor outside the individual. Rather, the whole idea of atomistic or clearly bounded individuals is challenged by the relationality of affect. Moreover, the capacity of bodies to affect and be affected varies between bodies and depends on the historical, political and cultural contexts involved. Consequently, affects may stick to some bodies, yet slide over others (Ahmed 2004b). We find this understanding useful for our thinking about the productivity and unpredictability of ailing encounters.

Second, we move on to examine how ailment can mobilise gendered, racialised and classed divisions of labour that extend from concrete encounters to the global scale. Although attending to ailment through care is demanding work requiring specific skills, historically, care and care work have been devalued as unskilled and underpaid work across the globe. Even though ailment is a shared human condition, the societal structures and organisation of care work specifically ail and affect those who have less power, influence and money. The long tradition of care research and theory has shed light on care work and the division of care labour (see, for example, Twigg 2000; Zechner and Anttonen 2022). We aim to add a new layer to this understanding through the concept of ailment. The concept of ailment enables an exploration of encounters and divisions around generalised care needs from the starting point that these encounters and divisions contain a possibility for care and support – but also a possibility for ignorance, harm and exploitation. Like ailing encounters, the divisions of care labour also include an affective dimension. The circulation of affects that stick to specific objects relates to how value and dignity are assigned to individuals and groups. The stickiness of affects and value is seen, for example, in the historical practices that have positioned working-class women and their bodies as dirty (Walkerdine 2011, 231), thus generating negative affects and valuations. These practices can also be seen today in connection to care workers and their bodies, many of whom are women, racialised and/or belong to the working class.

Affective encounters and caregiver ailment

In this section we explore ailment in more detail in the embodied encounters of (mainly but not exclusively) long-term care. In the vocabulary of Main (1957), the ailment of an individual is always productive, in that ailment also affects and ails those who attend to it. We draw empirical examples from our own research, as well as research by others, to illustrate experiences and dynamics of what we, in the line of Main's work, call caregiver ailment. Main (1957, 140) used the term 'staff ailment' to refer to 'the distress suffered by patients' attendants'. Similarly, caregiver ailment refers to the experiences, dynamics and affects that ailment mobilises in embodied encounters between human beings. According to the understanding of ailment in this book, ailment is a social force that mobilises thoughts, emotions, affects, actions, omissions, happenings, institutions and more.

One of the most significant responses that ailment can mobilise in embodied encounters is care. Care researchers have shown that care is a particular kind of practice, a practice based on what researchers have called the rationality of care (Wærness 1984), sentient activity (Mason 1996) or, more recently, the logic of care (Mol 2008). The rationality or logic of care refers to the fact that responding to ailment with care requires situated knowledge that can change unexpectedly and is embedded in a human relationship (Fisher and Tronto 1990; Anttonen and Zechner 2011). Due to the unpredictability of ailment, responding to it in line with the logic of care requires sensitivity and the ability to respond to changing situations. Care is also always about a human relationship, in which the response of the recipient of care also plays an important role (Fisher and Tronto 1990; Valokivi and Zechner 2009).

Attending to ailment as a practice is dynamic and open-ended. Ailing is an active process that draws attention to the rapidly and sometimes unexpectedly changing nature of the human condition. An ailing body requires attention, but what the body requires today might change tomorrow – also depending on the attention that it receives today. In intimate family relations, a first sign of a care need may be a sense that something is not quite right, especially in the case of dementia or other illnesses without significant physical symptoms. As Spielman (1997, 812) notes, ailment is not only ' "an acute specific disease" but something harder to define, something pervasive (insidious, perhaps) yet debilitating and causing distress'.

In Liina Sointu's research (2018) about the affective practice of caring in spousal caregivers' stories of how they became caregivers for their partners with dementia, it was not at first clear that the other partner was in need of care. Partners who later became caregivers felt odd, worried or irritated – some of them even contemplated divorce because they felt so deeply disappointed or betrayed by their partners. When, however, it became evident that it was in fact illness that was bothering their partners, they felt it easier to respond. This was also related to the dynamics of a couple relationship characterised in Finland by the idea that adults should mind their own business. Ailment disrupts this balance and demands that caregivers occasionally act against their partners' own wishes. Before confirmation that their partners were in fact ill, caregivers found it difficult to help because this questioned their partners' authority and autonomy regarding their own lives, for example if there was a need for a doctor's appointment or if driving the car was no longer safe. Confirmation of a partner's illness was a turning point in their narratives, after which they acquired the moral position of a caregiver who, through their own embodied presence, provided security for their partner. This meant in practice that they began to conceal their own emotional states from their partners. Instead, they aimed at using a gentle voice and expressing patience through their embodied gestures in the presence of their partners. This example demonstrates how ailment shapes the ways in which people relate to each other and thus produces new moral positions and identities. Occasionally, the caregiver's own health and safety are in danger in ailing encounters. We will return to this aspect of caregiver ailment in paid and formal care situations towards the end of this section, but here we concentrate on informal care.

Care work in the services is often defined as formal care, and the care work performed by family members and other close ones as informal care. Informal care is generally accessed through existing social relations, whether parents, siblings or friends. While informal care is often perceived as being cost effective at a societal level, it is not cost free to individuals. Research has demonstrated that the costs of caring for an ageing family member may include lost income due to having reduced working hours to accommodate caregiving (Evandrou et al 2002; Henz 2006; Lilly et al 2007; Lee and Tang 2013; Van Houtven et al 2013), may come with negative health effects and have a negative impact on subjective well-being (Vitaliano et al 2003; Coe and Van Houtven 2009; Chen et al 2019), and may have an effect on family life (for example Bauer and Sousa-Poza 2015; Sointu 2018). Ample research has evidenced that informal caregiving for a spouse can cause prolonged stress, strain and health problems for the caregiver (see, for example, Son et al 2007 for a review), including lower self-reported health and a neglect of self-care (for example Teel and Press 1999). According to research comparing older-age spousal caregivers with non-caring older-age adults, those caring for an ailing spouse had a higher mortality than those without such caregiving roles (Schulz and Beach 1999). Gerontological research commonly applies the terms caregiver stress and caregiver strain to describe the negative effects that caregiving and care work can cause. However, caregiver ailment is a broader term emphasising the variety of affects that ailment produces in caregivers.

Caregiving affects caregivers' well-being indirectly by making it more difficult for caregivers to take care of their own basic needs, such as sleep (Sacco et al 2018). Both the caregivers' and care receivers' safety may also be in danger more directly because of the unpredictability of ailment. Illnesses such as dementia or other neuropsychiatric conditions may cause safety hazards at home. In Sointu's (2011) study about the everyday lives of wives who provided long-term care for their partners at home, staying awake and alert was an important dimension of their everyday (and night) lives. In the evenings they had to, for example, stay awake as long as their partners to prevent a fire from a cigarette. Sometimes their partners felt confused, suspicious or aggressive due to changes in their perception of the world because of dementia, and acted in ways that put the caregiver in jeopardy. Näre's (2012) research on informally paid migrant elder care workers in private households in Naples, Italy, revealed that live-in elder care work was characteristically intimate labour that could even involve the caregiver sharing the same bed with the ailing older adult (see also Näre and Diatlova 2020). In these cases, caregivers often had to renounce their normal sleep to attend to the ailments of their employers.

Sometimes a care receiver's ailment may manifest as violent outbursts that physically hurt and put caregivers in danger. Harmful or abusive behaviours may have been part of the relationship for a long time, or they may arise as part of the care receiver's illness (Isham et al 2020). Whenever aggression and violence coexist with care, ailment may demand a careful manoeuvring in everyday interaction, so as not to escalate matters into aggression and attacks (Kelly 2017; Vaittinen 2019). In the worst cases, caregivers may be severely hurt or even die (see Simplican 2015). Indeed, sometimes responding to ailment requires 'caring self-protection', by which Vaittinen (2019) refers to the everyday tactics that nurses had developed as part of their work at a nursing home. In situations where the care receivers were aggressive towards their caregivers, the nurses used these tactics to protect themselves, while simultaneously protecting the care receivers from being hurt in the violent situation. In this way they ensured that intimate care could be given despite the aggression, and that the situation would not lead to a neglect of care needs, that is, another form of violence.

Sometimes, a caregiver ailment manifests itself as caregivers' responses and actions, and in feelings of being afraid that they might hurt the care receiver. Previous examples illustrate how ailing encounters – as in all human relationships – involve power dynamics. Becoming a caregiver also means entering into a hierarchical position in relation to the care receiver. The caregiver is often (although not always) more physically, emotionally and socially capable of caring, but also of hurting the care receiver. Individual caring situations are indirectly affected by a complex network and history of care relations. This is particularly true in the case of informal care in which intimate family histories provide the context for care. If in the history of the relationship there has been violence by the care receiver, then becoming a caregiver provides an opportunity for revenge (see Sointu 2018). The growing intensity of care needs thus increases the risk of violence in a care relationship (Beach et al 2005).

The conditions that mobilise caregiver ailment are never isolated encounters between the caregiver and the care receiver. In contrast, these relationships are always embedded in broader societal structures and systems. If a caregiver ends up neglecting or sacrificing their own health and well-being, or otherwise ends up getting hurt, in the process of caring for their intimate other, there is always a third party involved (see also Banerjee et al 2012). This third party consists of all the actors – for example social policies and political authorities, institutional care providers, community members and so forth – who engender caregiver ailment by *not responding* to the care needs of the care receiver, by allocating the responsibility of care to the individual caregiver, and, finally, by ignoring their ailments. This is well illustrated by the dramatic growth of violent experiences and the perceived threat of violence seen among formal care workers in Finland. In 2005, 20 per cent of Finnish care workers in residential elderly care settings felt that they were 'subjected to physical violence or threats by care recipients or their relatives' on a daily or weekly basis (Kröger et al 2018, 60). In 2015 this had risen to 40 per cent (Kröger et al 2018, 60). This dramatic growth is no coincidence and has been systematically driven by the Finnish care policy, which has emphasised home care and independent living, and made it harder for older people to access residential care. When they do eventually access residential care, their care needs are already highly demanding. In Finland the coverage and resources (that is, staff levels) of formal elder care services has not kept up with the dramatic growth in care needs of the care receivers (Mielikäinen and Kuronen 2018), and one of the results is caregiver ailment.

A further example of the various forms in which caregiver ailment can manifest itself in formal and paid care comes from Lena Näre's ethnographic fieldwork, which included participant observation and aiding the nurses in their care activities in a dementia ward of a municipal care home in Helsinki in 2013. On the first day of her fieldwork, the ward nurse gave Näre a tour around the ward and introduced the various technological innovations in place that were meant to help in the daily care work practices. These included what the ward nurse called 'smart floors' in residents' rooms, in other words floors equipped with sensors that monitored and tracked movement in the room when the nurse was not present. When a resident set their foot on the smart floor, an alarm lit above the door of the room and on portable buzzers that nurses were supposed to carry with them at all times. One of the first observations Näre made in the ward was that instead of carrying the rather clumsy buzzers, the nurses left them on side tables and counters in the shared living and dining room. Left on their own, the devices repeatedly buzzed and moved on the table tops. Unused to the sound of an alarm each time the device began buzzing, Näre became anxious, stopped helping out with the kitchen chores or other activities, and sought a nurse to inquire whether someone should go and help out in the room from which the alarm was coming. Her anxiety was not shared by the nurses, who usually explained away the alarm as having been caused either by a cleaner, or by a resident who would call for help in an attention-seeking fashion. So, although the buzzers are intended to prevent further ailments of residents, such as falling out of bed, in a dementia ward with chronic staff shortages, it is impossible for the caregivers to respond to all potential ailments, many of which occur simultaneously. Similarly, Sidsel Lond Grosen and Agnete Meldgaard Hansen (2021) find that the sensor floors fragment care as the audible presence of mobile devices disrupts situated care practices and adds to the intensification of care work.

Caregivers are often assumed to be strong workers who work out of love and with a sense of vocation. This assumption often holds at least some validity – the whole idea of caregiving assumes that caregivers have strengths and abilities with which they can respond to the ailments of care receivers. Yet, attending to ailment through care is often both a mental and physical strain, whether it is done professionally or informally, paid or unpaid. Caregiving is, just like ailment, relational. Yet people who perform care work are not always recognised as ailing individuals themselves. Some of the straining aspects of care work remain hidden from the public eye because they are generally associated with negative affects. Care work and nursing can be seen as 'dirty work', involving dealing with aspects of humanity that tend to be shameful, such as excrement (Twigg 2000, 144–6; Isaksen 2002). Culturally, this work is expected to be performed silently and without attention being drawn to it. Nevertheless, those doing 'dirty work' have various ways of finding dignity in their daily jobs (Stacey 2005). To many care workers, the ability to endure, manage and survive through mentally and physically difficult working conditions, and the ability to serve ailing individuals even in conditions of drastic under-resourcing, can be important sources of pride and prestige – even when this prestige is not recognised by the wider society (Stacey 2005; Olakivi 2017). To other care workers, however, the same elements of care work – including drastic under-resourcing – are reasons to quit their jobs (Olakivi et al 2021; Van Aerschot et al 2021). Yet people can have unequal opportunities to quit their jobs, and sometimes care workers manage in ailing working contexts because they have limited alternatives due, for example, to age, gender and racial discrimination in the labour market (Näre 2013a; 2013b; Wrede and Näre 2013). In the following section, we turn to such unequal divisions of care labour.

Ailment in intersectional and global divisions of labour

How responding to ailment is organised in society also reflects the ways in which the citizen and the individual are conceptualised. Feminist care ethics and disability studies have long criticised the idea of the citizen and individual in dominant (neo)liberal political theory as a rational and unencumbered bearer of rights, which overlooks 'the material, relational and affective conditions on which the emergence and sustenance of the citizen depends' (Dodds 2007, 502). Importantly and somewhat paradoxically, the (neo)liberal paradigm of the atomistic individual-citizen promotes the articulation of social policies that depend on the availability of women as informal carers, despite often being articulated as gender neutral (see, for example, Dodds 2005).

The division of caregiving has been, and still is, unequal. It tends to follow the lines of other inequalities so that those groups of people, locally and globally, who are in less powerful positions are assigned the task of care (Daly and Rake 2003; Kittay 2005; Folbre 2017). Moreover, care is often provided with too few resources (for example England et al 2002; Leinonen 2009). As a result, those who attend to the ailment of others are at great risk of facing bodily and mental ailments of their own – a phenomenon we have discussed as *caregiver ailment*. This increasingly burdens people who are already in less powerful positions in society. Globally, women are most directly affected by ailment, as responding to ailment almost universally continues to be a woman's task.

Societal divisions of labour are often justified and legitimated by ideological and discursive structures that make them seem inevitable, natural or beneficial to all involved actors – and thus alleviate the distressing, bothering and troubling facts of inequality, such as the sedatives that alleviated nurses' distress in Main's (1957) study. Attending to ailment through care was long understood as the natural task of women, while actual productive work was performed by men. The care work that has been assigned to women – looking after children, chronically ill people, persons with disabilities, and older adults – diminishes their opportunities to participate equally in other societal activities, such as studying, politics and salaried employment (Wærness 1984). When care is defined as work, instead of something naturally feminine like motherhood (Wærness and Ringen 1987), it becomes clear that the division of care labour can be distributed in various ways (Leira 1993).

Fairly early on, the naturalness of care work as a women's task was questioned in the Nordic countries, and formal public services were developed in order to respond to the care needs generated by ailment. The Nordic welfare state has been called 'women friendly', since through public investments in paid care, it has offered paid work and steady income for care professionals, most of whom continue to be women (Peterson 2011; Karsio et al 2020). The development of the Nordic welfare state and the professionalisation of care work are interconnected (Evertsson 2000). Gradually, care work education became integrated into the national education systems, and expectations of formal competence rose (Wrede et al 2008). At present, Finnish care workers have the highest educational levels across the Nordic countries (Van Aerschot et al 2021). However, the Nordic care sector faces constant political demands, driving the lowering of formal education requirements in the name of entrepreneurial flexibility, economic austerity, and other neoliberal arguments. The reputation of the Nordic welfare state as being 'women friendly' has also been seriously harmed by the severe under-resourcing of paid care work since the 1990s (Wrede et al 2008; Hansen et al 2021).

Nevertheless, in the Nordic region, as well as in most other countries, the major share of elder care is provided informally, that is, by family and friends, and is not visible in social statistics (Kemper et al 2005; Bettio and Veraschagina 2010; Zigante 2018). It is estimated that as much as 80 per cent of all care in Europe is provided by informal caregivers, and of those caregivers, approximately two thirds are women who care as daughters(-in-law) and/or as wives/partners (Hoffmann and Rodrigues 2010). Some changes, however, are visible in the gendered division. In Finland, 50 per cent of those spousal informal carers doing care work with the support of informal care allowance are men (Sotkanet 2020). In the future, informal care is likely to become even more important due to ageing societies, cost-containment pressures, and austerity measures that favour informal care arrangements, which are perceived as being less expensive than home-based or institutional formal care (Zigante 2018). Furthermore, by supporting informalisation, care policies inherently define attending to ailment as a private matter that families should address among themselves (see Chapters two and three; also Karsio et al 2020).

In addition to gendered divisions of labour, intersecting hierarchies based on class, race and ethnicity have structured care work as a response to ailment (Duffy 2007). Domestic servants in the United States, for example, have often been, and continue to be, women of colour, in their white employers' households (Rollins 1985). While some of the care work earlier carried out in homes is currently performed within formal institutions, racial-ethnic women still have a central role in these services (Glenn 1992; Duffy 2007; Brodin and Peterson 2020). Dorothy Roberts (1997) describes this racialised hierarchy of labour as the division between spiritual work, done more by white women, and the menial work of racial-ethnic women.

Today, responses to human ailment are increasingly global. In the field of elder care, employers in both public and private sectors (including households) have looked for a migrant workforce either from the global labour markets or from already settled migrants, and often from racialised minorities (for example Shutes and Chiatti 2012; Wrede and Näre 2013; Olakivi and Wrede 2021). In southern Europe, migrant care workers tend to work in the homes of older adults since the availability of elder care services is scant. In northern Europe, migrant care workers are common in formal services, especially in urban areas. In England in 2017, one in five social care workers were non-British citizens (Skills for Care 2019). Many migrant care workers are disadvantaged by being migrants, but also by being from an ethnic and racialised minority, and by being women doing undervalued and low-paid care work (Christensen and Manthrope 2016). In the United Kingdom, foreign-born workers are more likely to work night shifts and in non-permanent jobs than workers born in the United Kingdom (Fernández-Reino and Rienzo 2019). Many of the British workers from black and minority ethnic groups may face similar issues as migrant care workers, including precarious and temporary work contracts (Hussein et al 2014). In contexts of under-resourcing, frontline care work is a source of such disadvantage. Out of all frontline long-term care workers in the United Kingdom, at least 10 to 13 per cent are likely to be paid under the legal minimum wage (Hussein 2017). Thus, responding to ailment is delegated to relatively marginalised people – as always seen in the history of care (Williams 2018).

By attracting care workers from poorer countries, ailing bodies in the affluent countries mobilise large-scale global phenomena (Vaittinen 2017). Again, this demonstrates how ailing bodies are not only dependent on others. Ailing bodies also create entirely new dependencies, including global chains of dependencies. By using the term 'global care chains', researchers refer to situations in which care-related migration – mostly women but increasingly also men – serves as a response to meeting the care needs in one country, and consequently contributes to care deficits in another country (Hochschild 2000; Parreñas 2001; Yeates 2009). The migration of an individual with care responsibilities always entails that care be redistributed and reconfigured anew, locally and across borders. Thus, global care chains are created around all forms of care, including child care and elder care as well as nursing in Asia, the United States and Europe (for example Lutz 2008; Yeates 2009; Isaksen 2010; Wrede and Näre 2013; Marchetti and Venturini 2014; Isaksen and Näre 2019; Huang et al 2021).

From the perspective of the country of origin, the need for care does not disappear with the person who has previously provided care. The migration of a family or kin member usually signifies a redistribution and reorganisation of both child and elder care responsibilities. Jessaca Leinaweaver (2010) discusses how the practice of child fostering enables Peruvian migrants to ensure care for their children and company for their parents, in a situation in which migration has left what she terms a *care slot* that needs to be filled. A care slot, referring to the family level, can be filled in various ways. For some care needs, people can find ways to respond from a distance (Baldassar et al 2007; Zechner 2008). Increasingly, the care slot (especially in relation to the care of ageing parents) is filled by commercial care services in middle-income countries such as Ghana (Coe 2017) and India (Lamb 2009), where informal care has previously been the norm. Migration is thus transforming what are considered as culturally acceptable ways to respond to ailment, including in the countries of origin.

In addition to individual families, global care chains can contribute to care deficits in entire countries and force economically underprivileged countries to manage with draining pools of care workers. According to the International Council of Nurses (ICN 2020), there is a shortage of nearly 6 million nurses in the world, which affects low- and middle-income countries the most, and currently approximately 3.5 million nurses are working in a country other than the one in which they were trained. The COVID-19 pandemic has furthermore revealed the dangers of nursing deficits in countries that export nurses abroad (ICN 2020). One of the largest nurse-labour exporting countries in the world is the Philippines. Over half of its approximately 10 million emigrant workers are women (Ellis 2016), and many have children and older relatives whose ailments need to be addressed in a different way after their emigration. In the case of young children, there is some evidence that fathers take over the traditional mother's task of child rearing (Lam and Yeoh 2018); however, less research has been done on the redistribution of labour in relation to elder care in Philippines.

Of course, ailing bodies in the affluent countries are not the only actors mobilising global care chains. Rather, global care chains are mobilised by affluent countries' inability to find adequate responses to the care needs of their ageing populations. In Finland, for instance, austerity politics in the context of elder care have made paid and formal care work increasingly precarious, burdensome, and ailment-intensive, and decreasingly attractive to Finland-born professionals (Kröger et al 2018; Olakivi et al 2021; Van Aerschot et al 2021). Currently, tens of thousands of educated care workers in Finland work outside the health and social services (although the estimations vary, see Virtanen 2018; Kuntatyönantajat 2019). Instead of investing in the working conditions to attract non-migrant workers, many employers have turned to global labour markets and/or migrant and racialised minorities to find a workforce that is willing – or forced – to work in precarious conditions (Näre 2013a; Wrede and Näre 2013). Thus, employers and governments in the affluent countries use migrant workers as proxy agents to respond to the ailments they themselves fail to address.

In public discourse, the global and domestic recruitment of migrants for care work in affluent countries is often presented as a practice that serves all of the actors involved (Näre and Nordberg 2016; Torres 2017; Lutz 2018). According to publicly circulating narratives, contemporary recruitment practices serve ageing populations' care needs in the affluent countries. They also serve gender equality in the affluent countries, as female-gendered care responsibilities are outsourced to migrant women (and men), enabling the labour market participation of non-migrant women beyond the increasingly unattractive and ailment-intensive care sector (see Isaksen 2010). Finally, these practices serve migrant job seekers' need for employment and income that their countries of origin fail to supply. Employment and income in turn enable migrant care workers to respond to their own and their family members' ailments, and the migrant care workers' remittances to their relatives in their countries of origin also serve these countries' national economies (Misra et al 2006).

To many citizens and institutions in the affluent countries, including recruitment agencies, the win–win narratives just described are both appealing and functional (Olakivi and Wrede 2021), in that few people want to appear as exploiters or people who benefit from the exploitation of others – and yet, these are the distressing, bothering and troubling identities that global care chains tend to construct for people in the affluent countries. To alleviate this distress and ailment, the win–win narratives thus ignore and obscure certain facts. Particularly, the win–win narratives of course ignore the long histories of economic and global inequalities rooted in colonialism and imperialism that make the labour market and living conditions in former colonising countries attractive to migrants from former colonised countries. Without global economic inequalities there would be no global care chains.

Instead of acknowledging global inequalities, the win–win narratives reinforce the public, phantasmatic belief in the existence of liberal, free and fair labour markets in which individual, capable agents can pursue – and achieve – their personal goals (Näre and Nordberg 2016). In this phantasy, there are no structural obstacles great enough to stop hard-working, capable and enterprising migrant workers from getting what they want, including a better life in a distant country. This appealing phantasy is of course not true and serves to mask the global hierarchies, inequalities and caregiver ailment inherent in global care chains. In the labour markets of the affluent countries, migrant workers face various obstacles that are often impossible to overcome, including legal structures that can disfranchise foreign educational qualifications. In the EU area, for instance, non-EU qualifications have little value, which makes many highly qualified non-EU migrants seek lower-level care jobs that require few formal qualifications (for example Adhikari and Melia 2015; Vartiainen 2019). To employers, these over-qualified care workers are relatively inexpensive labour. Due to various forms of structural racism and xenophobia in care services, foreign-born care workers also tend to have relatively disadvantaged opportunities in career progression (Doyle and Timonen 2010; Dahle and Seeberg 2013; Näre 2013a; Vartiainen 2019). In the Finnish care services, for example, the number of foreign-born care workers in managerial positions is close to zero (Statistics Finland 2020). The exploitation of migrant care workers in the most arduous and precarious care jobs reinforces their caregiver ailment and diminishes their possibilities to support their families and further respond to their ailments.

A clear loser in the mollifying win–win narratives is the political incentive to work for a better world for both migrant and non–migrant care workers, and the recipients of care (Olakivi and Wrede 2021). The recruitment of international migrants or other marginalised actors for care work in affluent countries can mask, but does not solve, the root problem: namely, the drastic under-resourcing and undervaluing of elder care work in the neoliberal framework of austerity politics that has made this work increasingly burdensome, ailment-intensive, and unattractive. Importantly, as Bridget Anderson (2015) points out, restricting international migration does not solve this problem either. What is needed is a new political framework in which the value of care and care work is recognised in national and international forums, and in which global and domestic inequalities are addressed in tandem.

FIVE

The politics of ailment

In this book, we have introduced ailment as a conceptual tool to analyse the ways in which societies have responded to ailment as a fundamental human condition. We have argued that while ailment is a productive and mobilising force in societies, its productivity should not be understood in a traditional capitalist sense because responding to ailment always includes unpredictability and a relationality that escape simple calculations. In this concluding chapter, we reflect on the implications of the complex dynamics that ailment produces and mobilises, and discuss the trends and possibilities of wider policy and market responses to ailment.

We suggest that taking the politics of ailment as a starting point when thinking about contemporary societies and welfare states requires a novel conception of humanity. We argue that it is time to change how humans are perceived, especially in social and care policies. The idea of a rational and economic profit-seeking *homo economicus*, the human that longs for market-based choices in care, should be consigned to the past. This is because such humans have in fact never existed, even though policy makers create policies based on these ideals. Hence, current policies attempt to reject the actual human: *homo aegrotus* – the ailing human.

Instead of ignoring the physical and mental frailty of all individuals and their ailment, *homo aegrotus* recognises them. The ailing nature of humans is understood as a permanent and all-encompassing feature in societies, and it empowers actions and creates webs of connections between individuals, families, communities, regions and countries. Ailment is simultaneously a decaying and renewing force, since the risks, vulnerabilities and precarity of all humans means that preventive, protective and caring actions are needed at all times and in all places. Thinking with ailment helps to make visible how this prospect of people's own ailment, or how the ailment of others, ails individuals, family members, citizens, and entire societies and economies.

When approaching the field of care with the concept of ailment, a new political regime becomes imaginable. This political regime derives from ailment in its two senses: the existential state of human ailing, and the affective or responsive state of being bothered by it. From this perspective, a large proportion of modern societies appears to be built around ailment. Ailment, thus, resides in the heart of society, creating networks of responses to different bothers. In these networks, some forms and bodies of ailment gain more attention than others. Consequently, in the forming hierarchies of ailment and in the struggles over their definition, the politics of ailment emerge.

As discussed in the preceding chapters, the last four decades have seen the rise of neoliberal economics and politics, which aim to subsume the whole of human life, and the human being in its entirety, into the service of capital accumulation and profit making on a global scale. In the context of ageing populations, this is especially visible in the elder care sector, which in welfare states is also directly connected to the role of the state in securing a politically defined level of care. The perspective of ailment here contributes to making more concrete and visible the political regime that emerges around neoliberal responses to ageing human bodies and populations.

Not only do specific needy and vulnerable groups, or specific care needs, become objects of market transactions, but the existential ailing nature of humanity becomes a site of capital accumulation, as ailment is responded to with practices of commodification, marketisation and financialisation. The ailing bodies of older people thus become sources of profit making, whereas the ailments of their caregivers largely remain misrecognised in the neoliberal regime.

Thinking about social and care policies with ailment

In Chapter two we reviewed the history of social and care policies in the western welfare states through the lens of ailment. We told the story of how ailment became recognised by the advanced welfare states, although ailment as a concept was never explicitly at the centre of developing social policies. We painted the historical continuum of sociopolitical responses to ailment with a broad brush, beginning from sanctions and very basic maintenance, towards acknowledging and governing ailment through welfare state policies, and finally to ailment as a market commodity, personal responsibility, and means for profit making. We also discussed how control, exclusion and profit making have been part of the historic response to ailment.

Prior to the development of modern welfare states, the response of society to ailment was sanctioning, together with the provision of some basic sustenance. The various forms of early poor relief were attempts to keep the most underprivileged individuals from dying – their *well-being* was not the aim, as that was the privilege of others. During the era of industrialisation, this goal was supplemented by the target of ensuring a sufficient, and sufficiently fit, labour force for the service of expanding capitalist forms of production. Therefore, social policies were expanded to (mostly) cover the needs of working men. Later, during and after the First and Second World Wars, the idea of social rights helped to create some of the first universalistic social policy systems covering the entire population. After a short period of increasing acknowledgement of ailment through public social and care policies, a new phase began in the history of ailment, where ailment increasingly became a site of, or means for, profit making.

Throughout history, social and care policies have readily been understood to concern the less privileged. The more privileged groups have had their needs covered typically privately and via exclusive insurance schemes, and so on. The ailment of groups and people categorised as particularly vulnerable have also bothered (ailed) those in power. Therefore, groups such as the poor or the disabled have been singled out as targets of sanctioning, punishing, stigmatising or caring policies and practices. Modern social policy systems have developed in different societies through various responses to the ailments of the poor and the working class, and as a means of controlling those groups. Yet, what has been concealed in these histories is that ailment defines the lives of *all* members of society – even elites ail, and their ailment, too, is a social force.

The Nordic welfare state has attempted to recognise the interdependencies between different social classes, and in part, therefore, its societal safety nets and welfare systems are more extensive than in many other countries. Indeed, a central argument for legitimising expansive public welfare services across political parties has been the idea of social cohesion and solidarity. It can be argued that an important dimension of solidarity is that the ailing of all classes, including the lower classes, is understood as a collective responsibility, wherein the ailing of the lower social classes affects, sticks to and ails also the higher social classes. Thus, reading the histories of modern social policy from the perspective of *homo aegrotus*, the ailing human, forces us to see that the social policy responses to the physical or economic ailments of the poor were at least partly responses to the relationally evoked ailments of the elite. Hence, the concept of ailment invites a subversive reading of the traditional understanding of the class system, and particularly the related and highly problematic metaphor of trickle-down economics in local and global scales. The subversive reading does not assume a social system in which the well-being of the prosperous groups trickles down to the disadvantaged and 'vulnerable'. Rather, this reading assumes a system in which ailment and the responses to it build up societies and social, political and economic entanglements. Ailment can hence be understood as a productive element, which forces and empowers states, societies, markets and individuals to respond. When based on the idea that all residents have the same social rights irrespective of class or market position, the universalistic social policies come closest to the recognition of the universal idea of all humans as ailing, and ailing as the element that binds people together and which potentially creates cohesion and solidarity between them. With the turn towards the marketisation of social and care policies, the responding to ailment as a democratic political project is being eroded as the productivity of ailment is directed towards marketisation and financialisation, and the human condition of ailment is subjected to serving the economic interests of financial (and market) actors that increasingly direct profits outside national economies and systems of taxation.

In sum, the sociopolitical context of ailment varies, and the possible responses to it depend on the historical and geographical context. Hence, not only individual care needs and individual responses vary, but the sociopolitical context of ailing defines what is recognised as a care need that requires a response, who should bear the responsibility for responding to the care need (nobody, family, private, public, third-sector or voluntary services and so on), on what terms (paid, unpaid, formally, informally, professionally and so on), and following what kind of practical logic (the logic of care or the logic of profit making).

Thinking about markets and financialisation with ailment

As we pointed out in Chapter three the needs of ailing and ageing bodies and minds do not easily translate into predefined products to be sold and purchased in the markets (Himmelweit 2007; Green and Lawson 2011). In order to respond to care needs in an adequate way, services must be organised following the logic of care, and not the logic of business and economics. The logic of care focuses on the needs of the individual, the care relationship and the sociopolitical context of ailing, while business activities are geared to making economic profit. Since needs for care are situational and temporal, they are seldom identical, even for individuals of the same age and with the same illness. Instead, care needs vary even for the same person at different times. This means that those attending to the care needs must organise their actions accordingly: that is, relationally, situationally and flexibly (Mol 2008). This is an uneasy fit with market logics that, on the production side, are based on pre-planned resources and products and the efficient use of labour, that is on calculations of output per unit of input. This leaves little room for the spontaneous changes that are inevitable in care.

Care is only one response among others to ailment. The politics of ailment is thus a wider field and concept than the politics of care. Care is often seen as a response to an individual's diminishing capacities, and the inability to be an economically productive member of society. Therefore, in capitalist economy, the organisation of care is defined as a burden that consumes resources. Thinking with ailment, care is not a burden. Care creates jobs, webs of meaningful connections and recently increasingly profitable business by way of marketised services and financial activities. The financialisation of care demonstrates the ability of ailing subjects to mobilise large-scale societal structures, including economic ones. The financialisation of care, however, also engenders a conflict between the actual care needs of ailing subjects, on the one hand, and the responses of financialised care services that recognise ailment only to the extent and in a form that the market can exploit it, on the other.

There are alternatives to these trends. Ailment opens up the opportunity to think about the political regime anew: how would it look and function if ailment was accepted and recognised on its own terms? At least it is obvious that the politics of ailment require concrete collective responses, since it has been shown that neoliberal, marketised and financialised arrangements of care that are based on the self-caring and self-investing subject are inadequate and have a tendency to increase inequalities (see Van Aerschot 2014; Andersson and Kvist 2015). Especially, older adults who have resources such as funds, assets, investment skills and social networks, may manage to organise their care in marketised and financialised systems of care. However, those with fewer resources will face difficulties.

Ailment, as a concept that is dynamic, offers an alternative to the neoliberal subject that is often treated as an object: something that needs to be activated and guided to become an independent, rational and self-caring actor. The prevailing policies that emphasise active and 'successful' ageing are examples of objectifying policies for care. These policies are also collective responses to ailment in that they are based on the mobilisation of individual and personal responsibilities through the *collective* stigmatisation of dependency and inactivity, and through techniques such as private insurance.

The ailing subject does not need to be activated since it is always already active: that is, bothered, concerned and preparing for their own as well as others' ailments, and capable of troubling, ailing and mobilising small- and large-scale political and economic structures. In the politics of care provision, marketisation as a tool and solution to ailment can function as a smokescreen for the welfare state to withdraw from the responsibility of responding to the ailment of populations (see also Hoppania 2018; Kröger 2019). Ailing, however, never stops and can never be fully contained. There is always a possibility of the (re)politicisation and democratisation of ailment and care policy.

Thinking about care work and global inequalities with ailment

Ailment disrupts the capitalist economy by presenting an entirely different starting point for thinking about society: the ailing human being. Capitalist logic considers human beings as productive only when they are able to work in paid labour. Thinking with ailment starts with the understanding of human beings as always productive in ways that go beyond productivity in the capitalist sense of the term: ailing subjects always mobilise *something*. The responses that ailment mobilises are not products, but relations and processes that may vary from care to neglect, from uneasy feelings to collective reactions channelled through care organisations, public policies and markets, to personal responses undertaken by the ailing person themself, their proximate family or a community member. What remains constant is the productivity of ailment.

Care and care work are the most concrete ways of responding to ailment in situated contexts of care needs. Without concrete responses to ailment, societies collapse. Responding to human ailment is the most central task in all societies. As we discussed in Chapter four, however, the responsibilities of concrete and embodied responses to ailment have been assumed as self-evident and natural tasks to be managed by marginalised actors, including (working-class) women, racialised minorities, and transnational migrants. In most contemporary societies, the societal status and monetary compensation for care workers do not reflect the importance of their work, and this relates to the present narrow and limited notion of productivity, which does not encompass care work as productive.

Instead, care work continues to be undervalued, hard, demanding and mostly under-resourced and underpaid work. Ailing subjects mobilise complex affects, including compassion and kindness, but also repulsion and disgust, and these affects tend to stick to those who work in close contact with ailment. Ailment, thus, troubles and bothers not only those who need care, but also the caregivers. This is what we have termed *caregiver ailment*. Contemporary societies cannot manage without care and care work. Yet, societies tend to marginalise and hide care work behind the closed doors of private households or in low-end jobs at the margins of the labour market, where the least visible actors of contemporary societies, including working-class women and racialised international migrants, perform the most crucial tasks of these societies. The concept of caregiver ailment emphasises also the fact that care workers are themselves ailing and have specific needs for healthy nutrition, sufficient breaks, free time, and physical and emotional safety.

Ailment also mobilises large-scale societal and political structures, money and of course people. When local and national responses to ailment fail, ailment can mobilise global care chains. Responses to ailment are thus becoming increasingly global. One thing, however, seems constant: societies' attempts to outsource responses to ailment to the most vulnerable people and societies. This misrecognition of the value of work needed to respond to ailment is accompanied by the fundamental non-recognition of *homo aegrotus*. Hence, responding to ailment continues to impact and ail women unequally. In countries with weak public welfare service provision, only the wealthiest women can outsource their duties to other women from a lower social class and/or migrant women. Yet, even in countries with developed public welfare services, women continue to carry the main responsibility for ailment in society, as informal caregivers, daughters, mothers, in-laws and paid care workers doing under-resourced and low-paid care work. Reimagining societies from the perspective of *homo aegrotus* would promote social equality between genders, classes, generations and societies at large.

The future of *homo aegrotus* and the ailing earth

The motivation to introduce ailment as a concept for care research and wider political thinking is also linked to the urgent task articulated by many environmentalists and climate change researchers of imagining and recreating society and inhabiting the earth in a way that is sustainable. As the Raqs Media Collective (2013, 113) has written, '[i]t is easy to mourn for an ailing earth. The more difficult, and interesting, task is to think of ways out of lamentation, or to imagine ways of living and inhabiting the earth that will not require us to commiserate with the future in advance.' The concept of ailment can be used to extend and tie the political discussion around care to environmental concerns. Some recent research strands and policy developments have already started to focus on how, for example, health is about interdependency, as in the idea of 'one health', which sees human, animal and environmental health as inseparably linked (for example Hitziger et al 2018). The discussions on the 'eco-welfare state', on the other hand, discuss the dependency of welfare states on the economic growth paradigm, and look for ways to bring together social and environmental sustainability (for example ORSI 2019).

The concept of ailment has the potential to further advance thinking and policies in these areas and to combine care theory and research insight into the debates (see also Williams 2018). Even if the welfare state policies that have benefitted many people have been built around, and affected by, the ailment of us humans, they have not been responsive to the ailment of the earth and the environment. But now that the earth is so clearly ailing and environmental catastrophe is on the doorstep, the shared condition with the planet needs a new vocabulary and analytical tools to map the way towards a more caring society. Earlier we wrote that without concrete responses to ailment, societies collapse. Likewise it is with the whole earth, and, indeed, some researchers are already talking about the beginning of planetary collapse (Gergis 2020). The ailing earth is implicated in the concept of ailment, through human interdependency with biodiversity and ecosystems, thus opening up possibilities for research and the development of sustainable, caring policies.

For humankind to continue to prosper on the globe, the *homo aegrotus*, the ailing human being, must be put at the centre of politics and policies, and this idea should be extended to the environment now and in the future. Welfare states can be governed and steered to respond to ailment: history demonstrates this. The much-criticised market forces have been restrained, controlled and boosted via social policies before, and they can be again in the future. In a world where the politics of ailment would guide political decision making, societies can be rebuilt on socially, ecologically and economically sustainable principles. The current global crises – the climate crisis, the COVID-19 pandemic and global economic inequalities – demonstrate that politics of ailment are needed more urgently than ever. We urge that attention is also paid to how ailment bothers and affects individuals, their own ailment and (prospective) care needs, and the ailment of others, even the ailment of the earth as seen in the current climate crisis.

The simple fact of an ageing population means concretely more aged bodies to look after and care for. This has been dramatically manifested during the COVID-19 pandemic, to which older adults have been seen to be especially vulnerable. The direct and indirect medical and health care responses produce significant economic activities, even if the pandemic also affects other parts of the economy by slowing down growth and production. The growth in activities has included, for example, the production of protective gear and medical equipment, while the field of tourism stagnated. This is what ailment emphasises in general, and not only in the case of epidemic viruses: that a large part of contemporary economies is built around ailment. The wider social and health care sector and the insurance sector also stem from ailment. Social and health care are thus not a strain on the economy, but an essential part of it.

Finally, what would the politics of ailment mean in practice? One recent suggestion comes from feminist economists in relation to the post-pandemic recovery programmes.

As countries around the world are developing recovery programmes to stimulate employment and the economy, it is not insignificant how these stimulus programmes are used. Jérôme De Henau and Susan Himmelweit (2021) have argued that these investments should be directed towards social infrastructures, namely towards building better child- and elder care services. They demonstrate that a care-led recovery programme would create more jobs while reducing gender inequality, compared to common construction-led recovery programmes. Investing in care and social infrastructures is also a much more environmentally friendly way to stimulate employment and the economy than investing in carbon-intensive industries. Ultimately, the post-pandemic world needs more caring economies and societies that recognise the fundaments of *homo aegrotus*.

References

Abel-Smith, B. (1992) 'The Beveridge Report: Its origins and outcomes', *International Social Security Review*, vol 45, no 1–2, pp 5–16, doi:10.1111/j.1468-246X.1992.tb00900.x.

Act on Social and Health Care Fees (734/1992) www.finlex.fi/fi/laki/ajantasa/1992/19920734 [accessed 28 October 2020].

Adhikari, R. and Melia, K. M. (2015) 'The (mis)management of migrant nurses in the UK: A sociological study', *Journal of Nursing Management*, vol 23, no 3, pp 359–67, doi:10.1111/jonm.12141.

Ahmed, S. (2004a) 'Affective economies', *Social Text*, vol 22, no 2, pp 117–39, doi:10.1215/01642472-22-2_79-117.

Ahmed, S. (2004b) *The Cultural Politics of Emotion*, Edinburgh: Edinburgh University Press.

Allan, S., Gousia, K. and Forder, J. (2021) 'Exploring differences between private and public prices in the English care homes market', *Health Economics, Policy and Law*, vol 16, no 2, pp 138–53, doi:10.1017/S1744133120000018.

Anderson, B. (2015) 'Migrant domestic workers: Good workers, poor slaves, new connections', *Social Politics: International Studies in Gender, State & Society*, vol 22, no 4, pp 636–52, doi:10.1093/sp/jxv040.

Andersson, K. and Kvist, E. (2015) 'The neoliberal turn and the marketization of care: The transformation of eldercare in Sweden', *European Journal of Women's Studies*, vol 22, no 3, pp 274–87, doi:10.1177/1350506814544912.

Annola, J. (2019) 'Maternalism and workhouse matrons in nineteenth-century Finland', *Women's History Review*, vol 28, no 6, pp 950–66, doi:10.1080/09612025.2018.1516243.

Anttonen, A. and Sipilä, J. (2000) *Suomalaista sosiaalipolitiikkaa* [Finnish Social Policy], Tampere: Vastapaino.

Anttonen, A. and Häikiö, L. (2011) 'Care "going market": Finnish elderly-care policies in transition', *Nordic Journal of Social Research*, vol 2, no 2, pp 70–90, doi:10.7577/njsr.2050.

Anttonen, A. and Zechner, M. (2011) 'Theorizing care and care work' in B. Pfau-Effinger and T. Rostgaard (eds) *Care Between Work and Welfare in European Societies*, Basingstoke: Palgrave Macmillan, pp 15–34.

Anttonen, A. and Meagher, G. (2013) 'Mapping marketisation: Concepts and goals' in G. Meagher and M. Szebehely (eds) *Marketisation in Nordic Eldercare: A Research Report on Legislation, Oversight, Extent and Consequences*, Stockholm: Stockholm University Press, pp 13–22.

Anttonen, A. and Karsio, O. (2017) 'How marketisation is changing the Nordic model of care for older people' in F. Martinelli, A. Anttonen and M. Mätzke (eds) *Social Services Disrupted: Changes, Challenges and Policy Implications for Europe in Times of Austerity*, Cheltenham: Edward Elgar, pp 219–38.

Anttonen, A., Häikiö, L. and Stefánsson, K. (eds) (2012) *Welfare State, Universalism and Diversity*, Cheltenham: Edward Elgar.

Bailey, D. (2015) 'The environmental paradox of the welfare state: The dynamics of sustainability', *New Political Economy*, vol 20, no 6, pp 793–811, doi:10.1080/13563467.2015.1079169.

Baldassar, L., Baldock, C. and Wilding, R. (2007) *Families Caring Across Borders: Migration, Ageing and Transnational Caregiving*, Basingstoke: Palgrave Macmillan.

Bambra, C. (2005) 'Cash versus services: "Worlds of welfare" and the decommodification of cash benefits and health care services', *Journal of Social Policy*, vol 34, no 2, pp 195–213, doi:10.1017/S0047279404008542.

Banerjee, A., Daly, T., Armstrong, P., Szebehely, M., Armstrong, H. and Lafrance, S. (2012) 'Structural violence in long-term, residential care for older people: Comparing Canada and Scandinavia', *Social Science & Medicine*, vol 74, no 3, pp 390–8, doi:10.1016/j.socscimed.2011.10.037.

Barad, K. (2007) *Meeting the Universe Halfway: Quantum Physics and the Entanglement of Matter and Meaning*, Durham: Duke University Press.

Bauer, J. M. and Sousa-Poza, A. (2015) 'Impacts of informal caregiving on caregiver: Employment, health, and family', *Journal of Population Ageing*, vol 8, no 3, pp 113–45, doi:10.1007/s12062-015-9116-0.

Beach, S. R., Schulz, R., Williamson, G. M., Miller, L. S., Weiner, M. F. and Lance, C. E. (2005) 'Risk factors for potentially harmful informal caregiver behavior', *Journal of American Geriatric Society*, vol 53, no 2, pp 255–61, doi:10.1111/j.1532-5415.2005.53111.x.

Beck, H. (ed) (1997) *The Origins of the Authoritarian Welfare state in Prussia. Conservatives, Bureaucracy and the Social Question 1815–70*, Ann Arbor: The University of Michigan Press.

Béland, D. and Mahon, R. (2016) *Advanced Introduction to Social Policy*, Cheltenham: Edward Elgar.

de la Bellacasa, M. P. (2012) ' "Nothing comes without its world": Thinking with care', *The Sociological Review*, vol 60, no 2, pp 197–216, doi:10.1111/j.1467-954X.2012.02070.x.

Bettio, F. and Verashchagina, A. (2010) *Long-term Care for the Elderly: Provisions and Providers in 33 European Countries*, Luxembourg: Publications office of the European Union.

Bernhard, S. (2010) 'From conflict to consensus: European neoliberalism and the debate on the future of EU social policy', *Work Organisation, Labour and Globalisation*, vol 4, no 1, pp 175–92, doi:10.13169/workorgalaboglob.4.1.0175.

Beveridge, W. (1942) *Social Insurance and Allied Services*, American edition, New York: The Macmillan Company.

Blackman, L. (2012) *Immaterial Bodies: Affect, Embodiment, Mediation*, London: Sage.

Blackman, L. (2015) 'Affective politics, debility and hearing voices: Towards a feminist politics of ordinary suffering', *Feminist Review*, vol 111, no 1, pp 25–41, doi:10.1057/fr.2015.24.

Bonoli, G. (1997) 'Classifying welfare states: A two-dimension approach', *Journal of Social Policy*, vol 26, no 3, pp 351–72, doi:10.1017/S0047279497005059.

Bottery, S. and Babalola, G. (2020) *Social care 360*, www.kingsfund. org.uk/sites/default/files/2020-05/Social%20care%20360%20 2020%20PDF_0.pdf [accessed 28 October 2020].

Braun, R. A., Kopecky, K. A. and Koreshkova, T. (2019) 'Old, frail, and uninsured: Accounting for features of the U.S. long-term care insurance market', *Econometrica*, vol 87, no 3, pp 981–1019, doi:10.3982/ECTA15295.

Brennan, D., Cass, B., Himmelweit, S. and Szebehely, M. (2012) 'The marketisation of care: Rationales and consequences in Nordic and liberal care regimes', *Journal of European Social Policy*, vol 22, no 4, pp 377–91, doi:10.1177/0958928712449772.

Briggs, A. (2006) 'The welfare state in historical perspective' in C. Pierson and F. G. Castles (eds) *The Welfare State Reader*, 2nd edition, Cambridge: Polity, pp 16–29.

Brodin, H. and Peterson, E. (2020) 'Equal opportunities? Gendering and racialising the politics of entrepreneurship in Swedish eldercare', *NORA – Nordic Journal of Feminist and Gender Research*, vol 28, no 2, pp 99–112, doi:10.1080/08038740.2019.1698653.

Brown, K. (2011) '"Vulnerability": Handle with care', *Ethics and Social Welfare*, vol 5, no 3, pp 313–21, doi:10.1080/ 17496535.2011.597165.

Brown, R., Carlson, B., Dale, S., Foster, L., Phillips, B. and Schore, J. (2007) *Cash and Counselling: Improving the Lives of Medic-aid Beneficiaries Who Need Personal Care or Home and Community-Based Services. Final Report*, Princeton: Mathematica Policy Research Inc.

Brunila, K. and Siivonen, P. (2016) 'Preoccupied with the self: Towards self-responsible, enterprising, flexible and self-centred subjectivity in education', *Discourse: Studies in the Cultural Politics of Education*, vol 37, no 1, pp 56–69, doi:10.1080/01596306.2014.927721.

Burns, D. J., Cowie, L., Earle, J., Folkman, P., Froud, J., Hyde, P., Johal, S., Jones, I. R., Killett, A. and Williams, K. (2016) *Where Does the Money Go? Financialised Chains and the Crisis in Residential Care*, CRESC Public Interest Report, March, https://humme dia.manchester.ac.uk/institutes/cresc/research/WDTMG%20FI NAL%20-01-3-2016.pdf [accessed 28 October 2020].

Campbell, J. C., Ikegami, N. and Gibson, M. J. (2010) 'Lessons from public long-term care insurance in Germany and Japan', *Health Affairs*, vol 29, no 1, pp 87–95, doi:10.1377/hlthaff.2009.0548.

Chen, L., Fan, H. and Chu, L. (2019) 'The hidden cost of informal care: An empirical study on female caregivers' subjective well-being', *Social Science & Medicine*, vol 224, pp 85–93, doi:10.1016/j.socscimed.2019.01.051.

Christensen, K. and Manthorpe, J. (2016) 'Personalised risk: New risk encounters facing migrant care workers', *Health, Risk & Society*, vol 18, no 3–4, pp 137–52, doi:10.1080/13698575.2016.1182628.

Clare, E. (2017) *Brilliant Imperfection. Grappling with Cure*, Durham: Duke University Press.

Clarke, J. (2006) 'Consumers, clients or citizens? Politics, policy and practice in the reform of social care', *European Societies*, vol 8, no 3, pp 423–42, doi:10.1080/14616690600821966.

Clarke, J., Newman, J., Smith, N., Vidler, E. and Westmarland, L. (2007) *Creating Citizen-Consumers: Changing Publics & Changing Public Services*, London: Sage.

Clough, P. T. (2008) 'The affective turn: Political economy, biomedia and bodies', *Theory, Culture & Society*, vol 25, no 1, pp 1–22, doi:10.1177/0263276407085156.

Coe, C. (2017) 'Transnational migration and the commodification of eldercare in urban Ghana', *Identities*, vol 24, no 5, pp 542–56, doi:10.1080/1070289X.2017.1346510.

Coe, N. B. and Van Houtven, C. H. (2009) 'Caring for mom and neglecting yourself? The health effects of caring for an elderly parent', *Health Economics*, vol 18, no 9, pp 991–1010, doi:10.1002/hec.1512.

Coronavirus Resource Center (2021) Johns Hopkins University & Medicine, https://coronavirus.jhu.edu/ [accessed 28 October 2021].

Crowther, M. A. (1981/2016) *The Workhouse System 1834–1929: The History of an English Social Institution*, London: Routledge.

Cuellar, A. E. and Wiener, J. M. (2000) 'Can social insurance for long-term care work? The experience of Germany', *Health Affairs*, vol 19, no 3, pp 8–25, doi:10.1377/hlthaff.19.3.8.

Cushen, J. and Thompson, P. (2016) 'Financialization and value: Why labour and the labour process still matter', *Work, Employment & Society*, vol 30, no 2, pp 352–65, doi:10.1177/0950017015617676.

Dahl, H. M. (2017) *Struggles in (Elderly) Care. A Feminist View*, London: Palgrave Macmillan.

Dahle, R. and Seeberg, M. L. (2013) ' "Does she speak Norwegian?": Ethnic dimensions of hierarchy in Norwegian health care workplaces', *Nordic Journal of Migration Research*, vol 3, no 2, pp 82–90, doi:10.2478/v10202-012-0018-4.

Daly, M. and Rake, K. (2003) *Gender and the Welfare State: Care, Work and Welfare in Europe and the USA*, Cambridge: Polity.

Dasen, V. (2015) 'Infirmitas or not? Short-statured persons in Ancient Greece' in C. Krötzl, K. Mustakallio and J. Kuuliala (eds) *Infirmity in Antiquity and the Middle Ages. Social and Cultural Approaches to Health, Weakness and Care*, New York: Routledge, pp 29–50.

Dodds, S. (2005) 'Gender, ageing and injustice: Social and political contexts of bioethics', *Journal of Medical Ethics*, vol 31, no 5, pp 295–98, doi:10.1136/jme.2003.006726.

Dodds, S. (2007) 'Depending on care: Recognition of vulnerability and the social contribution of care provision', *Bioethics*, vol 21, no 9, 500–10, doi:10.1111/j.1467-8519.2007.00595.x.

Doyle, M. and Timonen, V. (2010) 'Obligations, ambitions, calculations: Migrant care workers' negotiation of work, career, and family responsibilities', *Social Politics*, vol 17, no 1, pp 29–52, doi:10.1093/sp/jxp026.

Downs, J. (2012) *Sick from Freedom: African-American Illness and Suffering during the Civil War and Reconstruction*, New York: Oxford University Press.

Duffy, M. (2007) 'Doing the dirty work. Gender, race, and reproductive labor in historical perspective', *Gender & Society*, vol 21, no 3, pp 313–36, doi:10.1177/0891243207300764.

Einiö, E., Wass, H. and Heinonen, M. (2018) 'Political exclusions attributable to poor relief in early twentieth-century Finland', *Population*, vol 73, no 1, pp 131–47, doi:10.3917/popu.1801.0137.

Eklund, M. and Markström, U. (2015) 'Outcomes of a freedom of choice reform in community mental health day center services', *Administration and Policy in Mental Health and Mental Health Services Research*, vol 42, no 6, pp 664–71, doi:10.1007/s10488-014-0601-1.

Ellis, H. (2016) *Global Care Chains: Addressing Unpaid Reproductive Labour in the Philippines*, Waterloo: International Migration Research Centre. Policy Points, Issue X.

England, P., Budig, M. and Folbre, N. (2002) 'Wages of virtue: The relative pay of care work', *Social Problems*, vol 49, no 4, pp 455–73, doi:10.1525/sp.2002.49.4.455.

Engster, D. (2019) 'Care ethics, dependency, and vulnerability', *Ethics and Social Welfare*, vol 13, no 2, pp 100–14, doi:10.1080/17496535.2018.1533029.

Erlandsson, S., Storm, P., Stranz, A., Szebehely, M. and Trydegård, G.-B. (2013) 'Marketising trends in Swedish eldercare: Competition, choice and calls for stricter regulation' in G. Meagher and M. Szebehely (eds) *Marketisation in Nordic Eldercare: A Research Report on legislation, Oversight, Extent and Consequences*, Stockholm: Stockholm University, pp 23–83.

Esping-Andersen, G. (1985) *Politics Against Markets*, Princeton: Princeton University Press.

Esping-Andersen, G. (1990) The Three Worlds of Welfare Capitalism, Princeton: Princeton University Press.

ETLA (2020) *Complementing Tax-financed Long-term Care with Private Insurance*, Etla Reports 98, https://www.etla.fi/julkaisut/yksityi nen-varautuminen-hoivan-rahoitusta-taydentamassa/ [accessed 26 February 2021].

European Commission (2018) *Peer Review on 'Germany's latest reforms of the long-term care system'*, https://ec.europa.eu/social/main.jsp?catId=89&furtherNews=yes&newsId=9008&langId=en [accessed 7 September 2020].

Evandrou, M., Glaser, K. and Henz, U. (2002) 'Multiple role occupancy in midlife: Balancing work and family life in Britain', *The Gerontologist*, vol 42, no 6, pp 781–89, doi:10.1093/geront/42.6.781.

Evertsson, L. (2000) 'The Swedish welfare state and the emergence of female welfare state occupations', *Gender, Work and Organization*, vol 7, no 4, pp 230–41, doi:10.1111/1468-0432.00111.

Fay, S. B. (1950) 'Bismarck's welfare state', *Current History*, vol 18, no 101, pp 1–7.

Fernández-Reino, M. and Rienzo, C. (2019) *Migrants in the UK labour market: An overview*, https://migrationobservatory.ox.ac.uk/resources/briefings/migrants-in-the-uk-labour-market-an-overview/ [accessed 14 April 2020].

Fine, M. and Davidson, B. (2018) 'The marketization of care: Global challenges and national responses in Australia', *Current Sociology*, vol 66, no 4, pp 503–16, doi:10.1177/0011392118765281.

Fine, M. and Tronto, J. (2020) 'Care goes viral: Care theory and research confront the global COVID-19 pandemic', *International Journal of Care and Caring*, vol 4, no 3, pp 301–9, doi:10.1332/239788220X15924188322978.

Fineman, M. A. (2008) 'The vulnerable subject: Anchoring equality in the human condition', *Yale Journal of Law and Feminism*, vol 20, no 1, pp 1–24.

Fineman, M. A. (2010) 'The vulnerable subject and the responsive state', *Emory Law Journal*, vol 60, no 2, pp 251–75.

Fineman, M. A. and Grear, A. (2013) 'Introduction: Vulnerability as heuristic: An invitation to future exploration' in M. A. Fineman and A. Grear (eds) *Vulnerability: Reflections on a New Ethical Foundation for Law and Politics*, London: Routledge, pp 1–27.

Fisher, B. and Tronto, J. (1990) 'Toward a feminist theory of caring' in E. K. Abel and M. K. Nelson (eds) *Circles of Care*, Albany: State University of New York Press, pp 35–62.

Folbre, N. (2017) 'The care penalty and gender inequality' in S. L. Averett, L. M. Argys and S. D. Hoffman (eds) *The Oxford Handbook of Women and the Economy*, New York: Oxford University Press, pp 1–20.

Forder, J., Jones, K., Glendinning, C., Caiels, J., Welch, E., Baxter, K., Davidson, J., Windle, K., Irvine, A., King, D. and Dolan, P. (2012) *Evaluation of the Personal Health Budget Pilot Programme. Final Report*, London: Department of Health.

Fuchs, S. and Offe, C. (2009) 'Welfare state formation in the enlarged European Union. Patterns of reform in postcommunist states' in C. Rumford (ed) *The Sage Handbook of European Studies*, Los Angeles: Sage, pp 420–41.

Gairdner, W. (2002) '"The Ailment"–45 years later', *Clinical Child Psychology and Psychiatry*, vol 7, no 2, pp 288–94, doi:10.1177/1359104502007002014.

Gergis, J. (2020) 'The great unravelling: "I never thought I'd live to see the horror of planetary collapse"', *The Guardian*, www.theguardian.com/australia-news/2020/oct/15/the-great-unravelling-i-never-thought-id-live-to-see-the-horror-of-planetary-collapse [accessed 30 October 2020].

Gilbert, N. (2002) *Transformation of the Welfare State. The Silent Surrender of Public Responsibility*, Oxford: Oxford University Press.

Gingrich, J. (2011) *Making Markets in the Welfare State*, Cambridge: Cambridge University Press.

Glasby, J., Zhang, Y., Bennett, M. R. and Hall, P. (2020) 'A lost decade? A renewed case for adult social care reform in England', *Journal of Social Policy*, vol 50, no 2, pp 1–32. doi:10.1017/S0047279420000288.

Glendinning, C., Challis, D., Fernandez, J-L., Jacobs, S., Jones, K., Knapp, M., Manthorpe, J., Moran, N., Netten, A., Stevens, M. and Wilberforce, M. (2008) *Evaluation of the Individual Budgets Pilot Programme. Summary Report*, York: University of York.

Glenn, N. E. (1992) 'From servitude to service work: Historical continuities in the racial division of paid reproductive labor', *Signs: Journal of Women in Culture and Society*, vol 18, no 1, pp 1–43. doi:10.1086/494777.

Gori, C. and Morciano, M. (2019) 'Cash-for-care payments in Europe: Changes in resource allocation', *Social Policy & Administration*, vol 53, no 4, 537–50, doi:10.1111/spol.12498.

Gough, I. (2008) 'European welfare states: Explanations and lessons for developing countries' in A. A. Dani and H. de Haan (eds) *Inclusive States: Social Policy and Structural Inequalities*, Washington: World Bank Publications, pp 39–72.

Gough, I. (2010) 'Economic crisis, climate change and the future of welfare states', *Twenty-First Century Society*, vol 5, no 1, 51–64, doi:10.1080/17450140903484049.

Gough, I. (2016) 'Welfare states and environmental states: A comparative analysis', *Environmental Politics*, vol 25, no 1, 24–47, doi:10.1080/09644016.2015.1074382.

Green, M. and Lawson, V. (2011) 'Recentring care: Interrogating the commodification of care', *Social & Cultural Geography*, vol 12, no 6, pp 639–54, doi:10.1080/14649365.2011.601262.

Greener, I. (2018) *Social Policy after the Financial Crisis. A Progressive Response*, Cheltenham: Edward Elgar Publishing.

Greve, B. (2014) *Historical Dictionary of the Welfare state*, 3rd edition, Lanham: Rowman & Littlefield.

Grosen, S. L. and Hansen, A. M. (2021) 'Sensor-floors: Changing work and values in care for frail older persons', *Science, Technology, & Human Values*, vol 46, no 2, pp 254–74, doi:10.1177/0162243920911959.

Ha, S. C., Kim, H. J. and Palmer, A. (2017) 'The relationship between public long-term care insurance awareness and preparation for later life in South Korea', *Journal of Social Service Research*, vol 43, no 4, pp 510–26, doi:10.1080/01488376.2017.1324829.

Halmekoski, J. (2011) *Orjamarkkinat: Huutolaislasten kohtaloita Suomessa* [Child Auctions: Stories of Auction Children in Finland], Helsinki: Gummerus.

Hansen, L., Dahl, H. M. and Horn, L. (eds) (2021) *A Care Crisis in the Nordic Welfare States – Care Work, Gender Equality and Welfare State Sustainability*, Bristol: Policy Press.

Harrington, C., Jacobsen, F. F., Panos, J., Pollock, A., Sutaria, S. and Szebehely, M. (2017) 'Marketization in long-term care: A cross-country comparison of large for-profit nursing home chains', *Health Services Insights*, vol 10, no 1, pp 1–23, doi:10.1177/1178632917710533.

Harry, M. L., Mahoney, K. J., Mahoney, E. K. and Shen, C. (2017) 'The Cash and Counseling model of self-directed long-term care: Effectiveness with young adults with disabilities', *Disability and Health Journal*, vol 10, no 4, pp 492–501, doi:10.1016/j.dhjo.2017.03.001.

Harvey, D. (2005) *A Brief History of Neoliberalism*, Oxford: Oxford University Press.

Hatton, C. and Waters, J. (2011) *The National Personal Budget Survey*, Lancaster: Lancaster University.

Hay, C. (2004) 'The normalizing role of rationalist assumptions in the institutional embedding of neoliberalism', *Economy and Society*, vol 33, no 4, pp 500–27, doi:10.1080/0308514042000285260.

Hedin, U.-C. and Månsson, S.-A. (2012) 'Whistleblowing processes in Swedish public organisations – complaints and consequences', *European Journal of Social Work*, vol 15, no 2, pp 151–67, doi:10.1080/13691457.2010.543890.

Hemerjick, A. C. (2012) 'Two or three waves of welfare state transformation?' in N. Morel, B. Palier and J. Palme (eds) *Towards a Social Investment Welfare State? Ideas, Policies and Challenges*, Bristol: Policy Press, pp 33–60.

De Henau, J. and Himmelweit, S. (2021) 'A care-led recovery from Covid-19: Investing in high-quality care to stimulate and rebalance the economy', *Feminist Economics*, vol 27, no 1–2, pp 453–69, doi:10.1080/13545701.2020.1845390.

Henz, U. (2006) 'Informal caregiving at working age: Effects of job characteristics and family configuration', *Journal of Marriage and Family*, vol 68, no 2, pp 411–29. doi:10.1111/j.1741-3737.2006.00261.x.

Hermann, C. (2014) 'Structural adjustment and neoliberal convergence in labour markets and welfare: The impact of the crisis and austerity measures on European economic and social models', *Competition & Change*, vol 18, no 2, pp 111–30, doi:10.1179/1024529414Z.00000000051.

Himmelweit, S. (2007) 'The prospects for caring: Economic theory and policy analysis', *Cambridge Journal of Economics*, vol 31, no 4, pp 581–99. doi:10.1093/cje/bem011.

Hitchcock, T. (1985) *The English Workhouse: A Study in Institutional Poor Relief in Selected Counties 1696–1750*, Oxford: University of Oxford.

Hitziger, M., Esposito, R., Canali, M., Aragrande, M., Häsler, B. and Rüegg, S. (2018) 'Knowledge integration in One Health policy formulation, implementation and evaluation', *Bulletin of the World Health Organization*, vol 96, no 3, pp 211–18, doi:10.2471/BLT.17.202705.

Hjelt, Y. (2019) 'Näin vanhusten hoivayhtiöt pyörittivät haamuhoitajajärjestelmää – Luottamusmies: "Kun työntekijä ei tule töihin, siinä säästetään sen palkka"' [This is how care companies operate, union steward says: when the care worker does not show up to work, the companies save money], The Finnish Broadcasting Company, 5 March, https://yle.fi/uutiset/3-10671 284 [accessed 15 April 2020].

Hochschild, A. R. (2000) *The Nanny Chain*, American Prospect, https://www.prospect.org/features/nanny-chain [accessed 31 October 2020].

Hoffmann, F. and Rodrigues, R. (2010) *Informal Carers: Who Takes Care of Them?* Policy brief, April, Vienna: European Centre for Social Welfare Policy and Research, https://www.euro.centre.org/publications/detail/387 [accessed 31 October 2021].

Hoppania, H.-K. (2015) *Care as a Site of Political Struggle*, Publications of the Department of Political and Economic Studies 25/2015, University of Helsinki, Helsinki: Unigrafia.

Hoppania, H.-K. (2018) 'Politicisation, engagement, depoliticisation – The neoliberal politics of care', *Critical Social Policy*, vol 39, no 2, pp 229–47, doi:10.1177/0261018318772032.

Hoppania, H.-K. and Vaittinen, T. (2015) 'A Household Full of Bodies: Neoliberalism, Care and "the Political"', *Global Society*, vol 29, no 1, pp 70–88, doi:10.1080/13600826.2014.974515.

Hoppania, H.-K., Karsio, O., Näre, L., Olakivi, A., Sointu, L., Vaittinen, T. and Zechner, M. (2016) *Hoivan arvoiset – Vaiva yhteiskunnan ytimessä* [Worthy of Care: Ailment in the Heart of the Society], Helsinki: Gaudeamus.

Hoppania, H.-K., Olakivi, A., Zechner, M. and Näre, L. (2021) 'Managerialism as a failing response to the care crisis' in L. L. Hansen, H. M. Dahl and L. Horn (eds) *A Care Crisis in the Women-friendly Nordic Welfare States*, Bristol: Policy Press, pp 109–30.

Hoppania, H.-K., Näre, L., Vaittinen, T., Zechner, M. and Karsio, O. (2022) 'Financialization of eldercare in a Nordic welfare state', *Journal of Social Policy*, vol 1, no 19, doi:10.1017/S0047279422000137.

Horton, A. (2022) 'Financialization and non-disposable women: Real estate, debt and labour in UK care homes', *Environment and Planning A: Economy and Space*, vol 54, no 1, pp 144–59, doi:10.1177/0308518X19862580.

Huang, S. S., Banaszak-Holl, J., Yuan, S. and Hirth, R. A. (2021) 'The determinants and variation of nursing home private-pay prices: Organizational and market structure', *Medical Care Research and Review*, vol 78, no 2, pp 173–80, doi:10.1177/1077558719857335.

Hudson, B. (2014) 'Dealing with market failure: A new dilemma in UK health and social care policy? Commentary', *Critical Social Policy*, vol 35, no 2, 281–92, doi:10.1177/0261018314563037.

Hussein, S. (2017) '"We don't do it for the money". The scale and reasons of poverty-pay among frontline long-term care workers in England', *Health & Social Care in the Community*, vol 25, no 6, pp 1817–26, doi:10.1111/hsc.12455.

Hussein, S., Manthorpe, J. and Ismail, M. (2014) 'Ethnicity at work: The case of British minority workers in the long-term care sector', *Equality, Diversity and Inclusion: An International Journal*, vol 33, no 2, pp 177–92, doi:10.1108/EDI-02-2013-0009.

ICN (2020) *COVID-19 and the International Supply of Nurses*, Report for the International Council of Nurses, www.icn.ch/system/files/documents/2020-07/COVID19_internationalsupplyofnurses_Report_FINAL.pdf [accessed 20 August 2020].

Ikegami, N. (2019) 'Financing long-term care: Lessons from Japan', *International Journal of Health Policy and Management*, vol 8, no 8, pp 462–66, doi:10.15171/ijhpm.2019.35.

Isaksen, L. W. (2002) 'Masculine dignity and the dirty body', *Nora: Nordic Journal of Women's Studies*, vol 10, no 3, pp 137–46, doi:10.1080/080387402321012162.

Isaksen, L. W. (ed) (2010) *Global Care Work: Gender and Migration in Nordic Societies*, Oslo: Nordic Academic Press.

Isaksen, L. W. and Näre, L. (2019) 'Local loops and micro-mobilities of care: Rethinking care in egalitarian contexts', *Journal of European Social Policy*, vol 29, no 5, pp 593–99, doi:10.1177/0958928719879669.

Isham, L., Bradbury-Jones, C. and Hewison, A. (2020) 'Female family carers' experiences of violent, abusive or harmful behaviour by the older person for whom they care: A case of epistemic injustice?', *Sociology of Health and Illness*, vol 42, no 1, pp 80–94, doi:10.1111/1467-9566.12986.

Jarret, T. (2019a) 'Adult social care: The Government's ongoing policy review and anticipated Green Paper (England)', *House of Commons Library*, commonslibrary.parliament.uk/research-briefings/cbp-8002 [accessed 31 October 2020].

Jarret, T. (2019b) 'Social care: Paying for care home places and domiciliary care (England)', *House of Commons Library Briefing Paper Number 1911*, commonslibrary.parliament.uk/research-briefings/sn01911 [accessed 31 October 2020].

Jessop, B. (1998) 'The rise of governance and the risks of failure: The case of economic development', *International Social Science Journal*, vol 50, no 155, pp 29–45, doi:10.1111/1468-2451.00107.

Johansson, H. and Hvinden, B. (2007) 'What do we mean by active citizenship?' in B. Hvinden and H. Johansson (eds) *Citizenship in Nordic Welfare States: Dynamics of Choice, Duties and Participation in a Changing Europe*, London: Routledge, pp 32–51.

Jönson, H. (2016) 'Framing scandalous nursing home care: What is the problem?', *Ageing & Society*, vol 46, no 2, 400–19, doi:10.1017/S0144686X14001287.

Julkunen, R. (2017) *Muuttuvat hyvinvointivaltiot. Eurooppalaiset hyvinvointivaltio reformoitavina* [Changing Welfare States: European Welfare States Reformed], Jyväskylä: SoPhi.

Karsio, O. and Anttonen, A. (2013) 'Marketisation of eldercare in Finland: Legal frames, outsourcing practices and the rapid growth of for-profit services' in G. Meagher and M. Szebehely (eds) *Marketisation in Nordic Eldercare: A Research Report on Legislation, Oversight, Extent and Consequences*, Stockholm: Stockholm University, pp 85–125.

Karsio, O., Näre, L., Olakivi, A., Sointu, L. and Zechner, M. (2020) 'Vanhuus, vaiva ja tasa-arvo' [Old age, ailment and equality] in J. Kantola, P. Koskinen Sandberg and H. Ylöstalo (eds) *Tasa-arvopolitiikan suunnanmuutoksia: Talouskriisistä tasa-arvon kriiseihin* [Changes in the Equality Politics: From Economic Crisis to the Crisis of Equality], Helsinki: Gaudeamus, pp 227–42.

Karisto, A., Takala, P. and Haapola, I. (1988) *Elintaso, elämäntapa ja sosiaalipoltiikka – Suomalaisen yhteiskunnan muutoksesta* [Standards of living, ways of life and social policy: about the changes in the Finnish Society], Helsinki: WSOY.

Kauhanen, A. and Riukula, K. (2019) 'Työmarkkinoiden eriytyminen ja tasa-arvo Suomessa' [Labour market segregation and equality in Finland] in M. Teräsaho and J. Närvi (eds) *Näkökulmia sukupuolten tasa-arvoon – Analyyseja Tasa-Arvobarometrista 2017* [Perspectives on gender equality – analyses of the Gender Equality Barometer 2017], Helsinki: Finnish Institute for Health and Welfare, pp 80–100, https://www.julkari.fi/handle/10024/137 765 [accessed 23 October 2021].

Kaye, S. H., Harrington, C. and LaPlante, M. P. (2009) 'Long-term care: Who gets it, who provides it, who pays, and how much?', *Health Affairs*, vol 29, no 1, pp 11–21, doi:10.1377/hlthaff.2009.0535.

Kelly, C. (2017) 'Care and violence through the lens of personal support workers', *International Journal of Care and Caring*, vol 1, no 1, pp 97–113, doi:10.1332/239788217X14866305589260.

Kemper, P., Komisar, H. L. and Alecxih, L. (2005) 'Long-term care over an uncertain future: What can current retirees expect?', *Inquiry*, vol 42, no 4, pp 335–50, doi:10.5034/inquiryjrnl_42.4.335.

Kestilä, L., Knape, N. and Hetemaa, T. (2019) 'Suomalaisten sosiaali- ja terveyspalvelujen käyttö tilastojen valossa' [Finish social and health care service use in light of statistics] in L. Kestilä and S. Karvonen (eds) *Suomalaisten hyvinvointi 2018* [Finish Welfare 2018], Helsinki: Finnish Institute for Health and Welfare, pp 188–206.

Kittay, E. F. (1999) *Love's Labor: Essays on Women, Equality and Dependency*, New York: Routledge.

Kittay, E. F. (2005) 'Dependency, difference and the global ethic of longterm care', *The Journal of Political Philosophy*, vol 13, no 4, pp 443–69, doi:10.1111/j.1467-9760.2005.00232.x.

Knickman, J. R. and Snell, E. K. (2002) 'The 2030 problem: Caring for aging baby boomers', *Health Service Research*, vol 7, no 4, pp 849–84.

Kolehmainen, M. and Juvonen, T. (2018) 'Introduction: Thinking with and through affective intimacies' in T. Juvonen and M. Kolehmainen (eds) *Affective Inequalities in Intimate Relationships*, London: Routledge, pp 1–15.

Korpi, W. (1989) 'Power, politics, and state autonomy in the development of social citizenship: Social rights during sickness in eighteen OECD countries since 1930', *American Sociological Review*, vol 54, no 3, pp 309–28.

Krippner, G. R. (2005) 'The financialization of the American economy', *Socio-economic Review*, vol 3, no 2, pp 173–208.

Kröger, T. (2019) 'Looking for the easy way out: Demographic panic and the twists and turns of long-term care policy in Finland' in T. Jing, S. Kuhnle, Y. Pan and S. Chen (eds) *Aging Welfare and Social Policy: China and the Nordic Countries in Comparative Perspective*, Cham: Springer, pp 91–104.

Kröger, T., Anttonen, A. and Sipilä, J. (2003) 'Social care in Finland: Stronger and weaker forms of universalism' in A. Anttonen, J. Baldock and J. Sipilä (eds) *The Young, the Old and the State. Social Care in Five Industrial Nations*, Cheltenham: Edward Elgar, pp 25–54.

Kröger, T., Van Aerschot, L. and Mathew Puthenparambil, J. (2018) *Hoivatyö muutoksessa: Suomalainen vanhustyö pohjoismaisessa vertailussa* [Care Work Is Changing: Finnish Old Age Care in the Nordic context], Jyväskylä: University of Jyväskylä.

Kröger, T., Mathew Puthenparambil, J. and Van Aerschot, L. (2019) 'Care poverty: Unmet care needs in a Nordic welfare state', *International Journal of Care and Caring*, vol 3, no 4, pp 485–500, doi:10.1332/239788219X15641291564296.

Kuntatyönantajat (2019) *Arvio muilla kuin koulutusalansa töissä työskentelevistä terveys- ja hyvinvointialan (sote) koulutuksen saaneista* [An estimate of personnel with health and welfare sector education working in other fields], https://www.kt.fi/sites/default/files/media/document/muilla-aloilla-tyoskenteleva-sote-henkilosto-2016-ja-2017.pdf [accessed 2 May 2022].

Kuuliala, J. (2015) 'Nobility, community and physical impairment in later medieval canonization processes' in C. Krötzl, K. Mustakallio and J. Kuuliala (eds) *Infirmity in Antiquity and the Middle Ages. Social and Cultural Approaches to Health, Weakness and Care*, New York: Routledge, pp 67–82.

Kuusi, P. (1964) *Social Policy for the Sixties: A Plan for Finland*, Helsinki: Finnish Social Policy Association.

Lam, T. and Yeoh, B. S. A. (2018) 'Migrant mothers, left-behind fathers: The negotiation of gender subjectivities in Indonesia and the Philippines', *Gender, Place & Culture*, vol 25, no 1, pp 104–17, doi:10.1080/0966369X.2016.1249349.

Lamb, S. E. (ed) (2009) *Aging and the Indian Diaspora: Cosmopolitan Families in India and Abroad*, Bloomington and Indianapolis: Indiana University Press.

Lee, Y. and Tang, F. (2013) 'More caregiving, less working: Caregiving roles and gender difference', *Journal of Applied Gerontology*, vol 34, no 4, pp 465–83, doi:10.1177/0733464813508649.

Leinaweaver, J. B. (2010) 'Outsourcing care: How Peruvian migrants meet transnational family obligations', *Latin American Perspectives*, vol 37, no 5, pp 67–87, doi:10.1177/0094582X10380222.

Leinonen, A. (2009) 'Hoivatyöntekijöiden muutostoiveiden topografia. Kannanottoja vanhuksen kohteluun, henkilöstöresursseihin ja ikääntymispolitiikkaan' [Topography of care workers desires for change. Statements to treatment of the elderly, resourcing of personnel and ageing policy], *Yhteiskuntapolitiikka*, vol 74, no 2, pp 132–48.

Leira, A. (1993) 'Concepts of care: Loving, thinking and doing' in J. Twigg (ed) *Informal Care in Europe. Proceedings of a Conference Held in York*, York: University of York, pp 23–39.

Leira, A. and Saraceno, C. (2006) 'Care: Actors, relationships, contexts', *Sosiologi I dag*, vol 36, no 3, pp 7-34.

Lilly, M., Laporte, A. and Coyte, P. C. (2007) 'Labor market work and home care's unpaid caregivers: A systematic review of labor force participation rates, predictors of labor market withdrawal, and hours of work', *The Milbank Quarterly*, vol 85, no 4, pp 641–90, doi:10.1111/j.1468-0009.2007.00504.x.

Lloyd, L., Banerjee, A., Harrington, C. and Szebehely, M. (2014) 'It is a scandal! Comparing the cause and consequences of nursing home media scandals in five countries', *International Journal of Sociology and Social Policy*, vol 34, no 1/2, pp 2–18, doi:10.1108/IJSSP-03-2013-0034.

Lundsgaard, J. (2005) *Consumer Direction and Choice in Long-Term Care for Older Persons, Including Payments for Informal Care: How Can it Help Improve Care Outcomes, Employment and Fiscal Sustainability?* OECD Health Working Papers, No. 20, Paris: OECD Publishing.

Luttinen, J. (2019) *'Miltä mielestä tuntui, ei arvaa kukkaan'. Sodan kuormittavuus ja kriisinkestävyys Iisalmen pitäjän kotitalouksissa 1800-luvun ensimmäisinä vuosikymmeninä* ['Nobody Knows How It Felt'. The Burden of War and Crisis Resilience in Iisalmi Parish Households in the First Decades of the 19th Century], Jyväskylä: University of Jyväskylä.

Lutz, H. (ed) (2008) *Migration and Domestic Work. A European Perspective to a Global theme*, London: Routledge.

Lutz, H. (2018) 'Care migration: the connectivity between care chains, care circulation and transnational social inequality', *Current Sociology*, vol 66, no 4, pp 577–89, doi:10.1177/0011392118765213.

Mackenzie, C., Rogers, W. and Dodds, S. (eds) (2014) *Vulnerability: New Essays in Ethics and Feminist Philosophy*. Oxford: Oxford University Press.

Madra, Y. M. and Adaman, F. (2013) 'Neoliberal reason and its forms: De-politicisation through economisation', *Antipode*, vol 46, no 3, pp 691–716, doi:10.1111/anti.12065.

Main, T. F. (1957) 'The ailment', *British Journal of Medical Psychology*, vol 30, pp 129–45, doi:10.1111/j.2044-8341.1957.tb01193.x.

Manderbacka, K., Arffman, M., Aalto, A.-M., Muuri, A., Kestilä, L. and Häkkinen, U. (2018) 'Eriarvoisuus somaattisten terveyspalvelujen saatavuudessa' [Inequality in the availability somatic health care services] in L. Kestilä and S. Karvonen (eds) *Suomalaisten Hyvinvointi 2018* [Wellbeing in Finland 2018], Helsinki: Finnish Institute for Health and Welfare, pp 207–15.

Marchetti, S. and Venturini, A. (2013) 'Mothers and grandmothers on the move: Labour mobility and the household strategies of Moldovan and Ukrainian migrant women in Italy', *International Migration*, vol 52, no 5, pp 111–26, doi:10.1111/imig.12131.

Marshall, T. H. (1950) *Citizenship and Social Class and Other Essays*, Cambridge: Cambridge University Press.

Mason, J. (1996) 'Gender, care and sensibility in family and kin relationships' in J. Holland and L. Adkins (eds) *Sex, Sensibility, and the Gendered Body*, Houndmills: Macmillan, pp 15–36.

Massumi, B. (1995) 'The autonomy of affect', *Cultural Critique*, vol 31, Autumn, pp 83–109, doi:10.2307/1354446.

Meagher, G. and Szebehely, M. (2010) *Private Financing of Elder Care in Sweden: Arguments For and Against*, Stockholm: Institute for Futures Studies, https://www.diva-portal.org/smash/record.jsf?pid=diva2%3A484054&dswid=9918 [accessed 15 October 2021].

Meagher, G. and Szebehely, M. (eds) (2013) *Marketisation in Nordic Eldercare: A Research Report on legislation, Oversight, extent and Consequences*, Stockholm: Stockholm University.

Merriam-Webster (2021) Ail, verb, https://www.merriam-webster.com/dictionary/ail [accessed 15 October 2021].

Mielikäinen, L. and Kuronen, R. (2018) *Kotihoito ja sosiaalihuollon laitos- ja asumispalvelut* [Homecare and Institutional and Residential Care Services in Social Care], Helsinki: Finnish Institute for Health and Welfare.

Miettinen, R. (2018) 'Vaivaiset ja työkyvyttömät uuden ajan alun maaseudulla' [Paupers and disabled in the countryside at the beginning of the new era] in R. Miettinen and E. Viitaniemi (eds) *Reunamailla. Tilattomat Länsi-Suomen maaseudulla 1600–1800* [On the Fringes. The Landless in the Countryside of Western Finland 1600–1800], Helsinki: SKS.

Misra, J., Woodring, J. and Merz, S. N. (2006) 'The globalization of care work: Neoliberal economic restructuring and migration policy', *Globalizations*, vol 3, no 3, pp 317–32, doi:10.1080/14747730600870035.

Moench, S. and Stender, S. (2020) 'Medi(long-term)care for All: A Look Into the Future of Long-Term Care Insurance—Part One', *Society of Actuaries*, www.soa.org/globalassets/assets/library/newsletters/in-public-interest/2020/march/itpi-2020-iss21-moench-stender.pdf [accessed 31 October 2020].

Mol, A. (2008) *The Logic of Care. Health and the Problem of Patient Choice*, London and New York: Routledge.

Morgan, F. and Zechner, M. (2022) 'Uncovering Familialism: Cash-for-Care Schemes in England and Finland'. *International Journal of Care and Caring*, doi.org/10.1332/239788221X16323394887310.

Moysés, S. J. and Soares, R. C. (2019) 'Planetary health in the Anthropocene', *Health Promotion International*, vol 34, Supplement_1, pp i28–i36, doi:10.1093/heapro/daz012.

Nadash, P., Doty, P. and von Schwanenflügel, M. (2018) 'The German long-term care insurance program: Evolution and recent developments', *The Gerontologist*, vol 58, no 3, pp 588–97, doi:10.1093/geront/gnx018.

Näre, L. (2012) 'Hoivatyön glokaaleilla markkinoilla: Filippiiniläisten sairaanhoitajien rekrytointi Suomeen jälkikolonialistisena käytäntönä' [In the glocal markets of care work: The recruitment of Filipino nurses to Finland as a post-colonial practice], *Sosiologia* [Journal of the Westermarck Society of Finnish Sociology], vol 49, no 3, pp 206–21.

Näre, L. (2013a) 'Ideal workers and suspects: Employers' politics of difference in the migrant division of care labour in Finland', *Nordic Journal of Migration Research*, vol 3, no 2, pp 72–81, doi:10.2478/v10202-012-0017-5.

Näre, L. (2013b) 'Migrancy, gender and social class in domestic and social care labour in Italy – An intersectional analysis of demand', *Journal of Ethnic and Migration Studies*, vol 39, no 4, pp 601–23, doi:10.1080/1369183X.2013.745238.

Näre, L. and Cleland Silva, T. (2021) 'The global bases of inequality regimes: The case of international nurse recruitment', *Equality, Diversity and Inclusion*, vol 40, no 5, pp 510–24, doi:10.1108/EDI-02-2020-0039.

Näre, L. and Diatlova, A. (2020) 'Ageing/body/sex/work – Migrant women negotiating intimacy and ageing in commercial sex and elder care work', *Sexualities*, online first, doi:10.1177/1363460720944590.

Näre, L. and Nordberg, C. (2016) 'Neoliberal postcolonialism in the media: Constructing Filipino nurse subjectivities in Finland', *European Journal of Cultural Studies*, vol 19, no 1, pp 16–32, doi:10.1177/1367549415585557.

Needham, C. (2014) 'Personalization: From day centres to community hubs?', *Critical Social Policy*, vol 34, no 1, pp 90–108, doi:10.1177/0261018313483492.

Netten, A., Jones, K., Knapp, M., Fernandez, J., Challis, D., Glendinning, C., Jacobs, S., Manthorpe, J., Moran, N., Stevens, M. and Wilberforce, M. (2012) 'Personalisation through individual budgets: Does it work and for whom?', *British Journal of Social Work*, vol 42, no 8, pp 1556–75, doi:10.1093/bjsw/bcr159.

Newman, J. and Clarke, J. (2009) *Publics, Politics and Power: Remaking the Public in Public Services*, London: Sage.

Newman, J. and Tonkens, E. (2011a) 'Active citizenship. Responsibility, choice and participation' in J. Newman and E. Tonkens (eds) *Participation, Responsibility and Choice. Summoning the Active Citizen in Western European Welfare States*, Amsterdam: Amsterdam University Press, pp 179–200.

Newman, J. and Tonkens, E. (2011b) 'Introduction' in J. Newman and E. Tonkens (eds) *Participation, Responsibility and Choice. Summoning the Active Citizen in Western European Welfare States*, Amsterdam: Amsterdam University Press, pp 9–28.

Newman, T. (2002) ' "Young carers" and disabled parents: Time for a change of direction?', *Disability & Society*, vol 17, no 6, pp 613–25, doi:10.1080/0968759022000010407.

Noddings, N. (1984) *Caring. A Feminine Approach to Ethics and Moral Education*, Berkeley: University of California Press.

OECD (2022) *Long-term care. Web pages covering the topic of elder care*, www.oecd.org/els/health-systems/long-term-care.htm [accessed 14 April 2022].

Offe, C. (1983) 'Competitive party democracy and the Keynesian welfare state: Factors of stability and disorganization', *Policy Sciences*, vol 15, no 3, pp 225–46, doi:10.1007/BF00136826.

Olakivi, A. (2017) 'Unmasking the enterprising nurse: Migrant care workers and the discursive mobilisation of productive professionals', *Sociology of Health & Illness*, vol 39, no 3, pp 428–42, doi:10.1111/1467-9566.12493.

Olakivi, A. and Wrede, S. (2021) 'Pragmatic inattention and win-win narratives: How Finnish eldercare managers make sense of foreign-born care workers' structural disadvantage?' in V. Horn, C. Schweppe, A. Böcker and M. Bruquetas-Callejo (eds), *The Global Old Age Care Industry: Tapping into Care Labour Across Borders*, Singapore: Palgrave Macmillan, pp 169–91.

Olakivi, A., Van Aerschot, L., Mathew Puthenparambil, J. and Kröger, T. (2021) 'Ylikuormitusta, lähijohtajan tuen puutetta vai vääränlaisia tehtäviä: Miksi yhä useammat vanhustyöntekijät harkitsevat työnsä lopettamista?' [Psychophysical overload, inadequate supervisor support or inappropriate tasks: Why are more and more care workers considering leaving their jobs?], *Yhteiskuntapolitiikka*, vol 86, no 2, pp 141–54.

Olesen, V., Schatzman, L., Droes, N., Hatton, D. and Chico, N. (1990) 'The mundane ailment and the physical self: Analysis of the social psychology of health and illness', *Social Science & Medicine*, vol 30, no 4, pp 449–55, doi:10.1016/0277-9536(90)90347-u.

Orloff, A. S. (1993) 'Gender and the social rights of citizenship: The comparative analysis of gender relations and welfare states', American Sociological Review, vol 58, no 3, pp 303–28, doi:10.2307/2095903.

ORSI (2019) *Web page of ORCHESTRATING TOGETHER towards Eco-Welfare State: Orchestrating for Systemic Impact (ORSI) project*, https://www.ecowelfare.fi/en [accessed 31 October 2020].

Ortiz-Ospina, E. and Roser, M. (2016) *Government Spending*, https://ourworldindata.org/government-spending [accessed 11 April 2022].

Óskarsdóttir, S. (2007) 'From active states to active citizenship? The impact of economic openness and transnational governance' in B. Hvinden and H. Johansson (eds) *Citizenship in Nordic Welfare States: Dynamics of Choice, Duties and Participation in a Changing Europe*, London: Routledge, pp 18–31.

Paju, E., Näre, L., Haikkola, L. and Krivonos, D. (2020) 'Human capitalisation in activation: Young people outside of employment and education in Finland', *European Journal of Cultural and Political Sociology*, vol 7, no 1, pp 7–28, doi:10.1080/23254823.2019.1689834.

Palier, B. (2010) *A Long Goodbye to Bismarck? The Politics of Welfare Reform in Continental Europe*, Amsterdam: Amsterdam University Press.

Parreñas, R. S. (2001) *Servants of Globalization: Migration and Domestic Work*, Stanford: Stanford University Press.

Peterson, E. (2011) *Beyond the 'Women-friendly' Welfare State: Framing Gender Inequality as a Policy Problem in Spanish and Swedish Politics of Care*, Madrid: University Complutense de Madrid, https://eprints.ucm.es/id/eprint/18170/1/T33524.pdf [accessed 13 October 2021].

Phillips, J. (2007) *Care*, Cambridge: Polity.

Pierson, P. (1994) *Dismantling the Welfare State*, Cambridge: Cambridge University Press.

Pierson, P. (2001) *New Politics of the Welfare State*, Oxford: Oxford University Press.

Pongsiri, M. J., Bickersteth, S., Colón, C., DeFries, R., Dhaliwal, M., Georgeson, L., Haines, A., Linou, N., Murray, V., Naeem, S., Small, R. and Ungvari, J. (2019) 'Planetary health: From concept to decisive action', *The Lancet Planetary Health*, vol 3, no 10, pp 402–4, doi:10.1016/S2542-5196(19)30190-1.

Powell, M. and Hewitt, M. (2002) *Welfare State and Welfare Change*, Buckingham: Open University Press.

Price, D. and Livsey, L. (2013) 'Financing Later Life: Pensions, Care, Housing Equity and the New Politics of Old Age' in G. Ramia, K. Farnsworth and Z. Irving (eds) *Analysis and Debate in Social Policy*, Bristol: Policy Press, pp 67–88.

Puar, J. (2017) *The Right to Maim. Debility, Capacity, Disability*, Durham: Duke University Press.

Ranci, C. and Pavolini, E. (eds) (2013) *Reforms in Long-Term Care Policies in Europe. Investigating Institutional Change and Social Impacts*, New York: Springer.

Raqs Media Collective (2013) 'Three and a half conversations with an eccentric planet', *Third Text*, vol 27, no 1, pp 108–14, doi:10.1080/09528822.2013.752233.

Reckendrees, A. (2020) 'Why did German early industrial capitalists suggest workers' pensions, arbitration boards and minimum wages?', *Jahrbuch für Wirtschaftsgeschichte / Economic History Yearbook*, vol 61, no 2, pp 351–76, doi:10.1515/jbwg-2020-0015.

Reckwitz, A. (2012) 'Affective spaces: A praxeological outlook', *Rethinking History*, vol 16, no 2, pp 241–58, doi:10.1080/13642529.2012.681193.

Reich, W. T. (1995) 'History of the notion of care' in W. T. Reich (ed) *Encyclopedia of Bioethics. Revised edition*, New York: Simon & Schuster Macmillan, pp 319–31.

Roberts, D. (1997) 'Spiritual and menial housework', *Yale Journal of Law and Feminism*, vol 9, no 51, pp 51–80.

Rollins, J. (1985) *Between Women: Domestics and their Employers*, Philadelphia: Temple University Press.

Rostgaard, T. (2006) 'Constructing the care consumer: Free choice of home care for the elderly in Denmark', *European Societies*, vol 8, no 3, pp 443–63, doi:10.1080/14616690600822048.

Rudge, T. (2009) 'Beyond caring? Discounting the differently known body', *Sociological Review*, vol 56, no 2, pp 233–48, doi:10.1111/j.1467-954X.2009.00825.x.

Ryvkina, R. V. (2010) 'The social ailments of Russian society as an object of sociological study', *Russian Social Science Review*, vol 51, no 3, pp 89–97, doi:10.1080/10611428.2010.11065394.

Sacco, L. B., Leineweber, C. and Platts, L. G. (2018) 'Informal care and sleep disturbance among caregivers in paid work: Longitudinal analyses from a large community-based Swedish cohort study', *Sleep*, vol 41, no 2, doi:10.1093/sleep/zsx198.

Schultz Lee, K. (2010) 'Gender, care work, and the complexity of family membership in Japan', *Gender & Society*, vol 24, no 5, pp 647–71, doi:10.1177/0891243210382903.

Schulz, R. and Beach, S. R. (1999) 'Caregiving as a risk factor for mortality', *JAMA*, vol 282, no 23, pp 2215–19, doi:10.1001/jama.282.23.2215.

Seeleib-Kaiser, M. (ed) (2008) *Welfare State Transformations. Comparative Perspectives*, Houndmills: Palgrave Macmillan.

Shutes, I. and Chiatti, C. (2012) 'Migrant labour and the marketisation of care for older people: The employment of migrant care workers by families and service providers', *Journal of European Social Policy*, vol 22, no 4, pp 392–405, doi:10.1177/0958928712449773.

Siivonen, P. and Brunila, K. (2014) 'The making of entrepreneurial subjectivity in adult education', *Studies in Continuing Education*, vol 36, no 2, pp 160–72, doi:10.1080/0158037X.2014.904776.

Simplican, S. C. (2015) 'Care, disability, and violence: Theorizing complex dependency in Eva Kittay and Judith Butler', *Hypatia*, vol 30, no 1, pp 217–33, doi:10.1111/hypa.12130.

Skills for Care (2019) *Being a Personal Assistant. A brochure*, www.skillsforcare.org.uk/Employing-your-own-care-and-support/Resources/Working-as-a-PA/1.-What-is-a-PA/Being-a-personal-assistant/Being-a-personal-assistant.pdf [accessed 31 October 2020].

Sointu, E. (2016) 'Discourse, affect and afflication', *The Sociological Review*, vol 64, no 2, pp 312–28, doi:10.1111/ 1467-954X.12334.

Sointu, L. (2011) 'Läsnäolo hoivan arjessa' [The Presence of Informal Care], *Janus*, vol 19, no 2, pp 158–73.

Sointu, L. (2018) 'Slipping into "that nurse's dress": Caring as affective practice in mixed-sex couples' relationships' in T. Juvonen and M. Kolehmainen (eds) *Affective Inequalities in Intimate Relationships*, London: Routledge, pp 95–108.

Sointu, L., Lehtonen, T.-K. and Häikiö, L. (2021) 'The public, the private and the changing expectations for everyday welfare services: The case of Finnish parents seeking private health care for their children', *Social Policy and Society*, vol 20, no 6, pp 232–46, doi:10.1017/S1474746420000287.

Son, J., Erno, A., Shea, D. G., Femia, E. E., Zarit, S. H. and Parris Stephens, M. A. (2007) 'The caregiver stress process and health outcomes', *Journal of Aging and Health*, vol 19, no 6, pp 871–87, doi:10.1177/0898264307308568.

Sotkanet (2020) *Statistical Information on Welfare and Health in Finland*, https://sotkanet.fi/sotkanet/en/index [accessed 31 October 2020].

Spielman, R. (1997) 'The 40th anniversary of the publication of The Ailment by TF Main', *Australian and New Zealand Journal of Psychiatry*, vol 31, no 6, pp 812–16, doi:10.3109/00048679709065505.

Spinoza, B. (1677/1982) *The Ethics and Selected Letters*, Indianapolis: Hackett Publishing Company.

Springer, S. (2020) 'Caring geographies: The COVID-19 interregnum and a return to mutual aid', *Dialogues in Human Geography*, vol 10, no 2, pp 112–15, doi:10.1177/2043820620931277.

Stacey, C. L. (2005) 'Finding dignity in dirty work: The constraints and rewards of low-wage home care labour', *Sociology of Health & Illness*, vol 27, no 6, pp 831–54.

Statistics Finland (2020) 'Labour statistics on foreign-born employees', available on request from https://www.stat.fi [accessed 31 October 2020].

Szebehely, M. (ed) (2003) *Hemhjälp i Norden: Illustrationer och reflektioner* [Home care in the Nordic Countries: Illustrations and reflections], Lund: Studentlitteratur.

Tamiya, N., Noguchi, H., Nishi, A., Reich, M. R., Ikegami, N., Hashimoto, H., Shibuya, K., Kawachi, I. and Campbell, J. C. (2011) 'Population ageing and wellbeing: Lessons from Japan's long-term care insurance policy', *Lancet*, vol 378, no 9797, pp 1183–92, doi:10.1016/S0140-6736(11)61176-8.

Teel, C. S. and Press, A. N. (1999) 'Fatigue among elders in caregiving and noncaregiving roles', *Western Journal of Nursing Research*, vol 21, no 4, pp 498–520, doi:10.1177/01939459922044009.

Tevameri, T. (2020) *Missä mennään sote-toimiala? Sosiaali- ja terveyspalveluiden Toimialaraportti* [Where Are We Now with the Health and Social Services Sector? Sector Report on Health and Social Services], Helsinki: The Ministry of Economic Affairs and Employment.

Tevameri, T. (2021) *Katsaus sote-alan työvoimaan. Toimintaympäristön ajankohtaisten muutosten ja pidemmän aikavälin tarkastelua* [Review of Labour Force in the Healthcare and Social Welfare Sector: Examination of the Operating Environment in the Light of the Current Changes and in the Longer Term], Helsinki: The Ministry of Economic Affairs and Employment.

The Care Collective (Chatzidakis, C., Hakim, J., Litter, J., Rottenberg, C. and Segal, L.) (2020) *The Care Manifesto. The Politics of Interdependence*, London, New York: Verso.

Theobald, H. (2012) 'Combining welfare mix and new public management: The case of long-term care insurance in Germany', *International Journal of Social Welfare*, vol 21, no 1, pp 61–74, doi:10.1111/j.1468-2397.2011.00865.x.

Timonen, V. (2016) *Beyond Successful and Active Ageing: A Theory of Model Ageing*, Bristol: Policy Press.

Titmuss, R. (1974) *Social Policy: An Introduction*, London: Allen and Unwin.

Torres, S. (2017) 'Fobbing care work unto "the Other" – What daily press reporting shows', *Sociologisk forskning*, vol 54, no 4, pp 319–22.

Tronto, J. (1993) *Moral Boundaries: A Political Argument for an Ethic of Care*, New York: Routledge.

Tronto, J. (2017) 'There is an alternative: Homines curans and the limits of neoliberalism', *International Journal of Care and Caring*, vol 1, no 1, pp 27–43, doi:10.1332/239788217X14866281687583.

Tronto, J. (2018) 'Care as a political concept' in N. Hirschmann and C. D. Stefano (eds) *Revisioning the Political: Feminist Reconstructions of Traditional Concepts in Western Political*, Boulder: Westview Press, pp 139–56.

Twigg, J. (2000) *Bathing. The Body and Community Care*, London & New York: Routledge.

UN (2017) *World Population Ageing. Department of Economic and Social Affairs*, New York: UN.

Ungerson, C. (ed) (1990) *Gender and Caring. Work and Welfare in Britain and Scandinavia*, New York: Harvester Wheatsheaf.

Ungerson, C. and Yeandle, S. (eds) (2007) *Cash for Care in Developed Welfare States*, Houndmills: Palgrave Macmillan.

Vabø, M. and Szebehely, M. (2012) 'A caring state for all older people?' in A. Anttonen, L. Häikiö and K. Stefánsson (eds) *Welfare State, Universalism and Diversity*, Cheltenham: Edward Elgar, pp 121–43.

Vaittinen, T. (2014) 'Reading global care chains as migrant trajectories: A theoretical framework for the understanding of structural change', *Women's Studies International Forum*, vol 47, part B, pp 191–202, doi:10.1016/j.wsif.2014.01.009.

Vaittinen, T. (2015) 'The power of the vulnerable body: A new political understanding of care', *International Feminist Journal of Politics*, vol 17, no 1, pp 100–18, doi:10.1080/14616742.2013.876301.

Vaittinen, T. (2017) *The Global Biopolitical Economy of Needs: Transnational Entanglements Between Ageing Finland and the Global Nurse Reserve of the Philippines*, Tampere: University of Tampere.

Vaittinen, T. (2019) 'Exposed to violence while caring: From caring self-protection to global health as conflict transformation' in T. Vaittinen and C. Confortini (eds) *Gender, Global Health and Violence: Feminist Perspectives on Peace and Disease*. London: Rowman & Littlefield, pp 227-50.

Vaittinen, T., Hoppania, H.-K. and Karsio, O. (2018) 'Marketization, commodification and privatization of care services' in J. Elias and A. Roberts (eds) *Handbook on the International Political Economy of Gender*, Cheltenham: Edward Elgar, pp 379–91.

Valokivi, H. and Zechner, M. (2009) 'Ristiriitainen omaishoiva – Läheisen auttamisesta kunnan palveluksi' [Contradictory informal care – From helping the close one to a municipal service] in A. Anttonen, H. Valokivi and M. Zechner (eds) *Hoiva –Tutkimus, politiikka ja arki* [Care – Research, Politics and Everyday life], Tampere: Vastapaino, pp 126–53.

Vamstad, J. (2016) 'Exit, voice and indifference – Older people as consumers of Swedish home care services', *Ageing and Society*, vol 36, no 10, pp 2163–81, doi:10.1017/S0144686X15000987.

Van Aerschot, L. (2014) *Vanhusten hoiva ja eriarvoisuus: Sosiaalisen ja taloudellisen taustan yhteys avun saamiseen ja palvelujen käyttöön* [Care of Older People and Inequality: How Socio-economic Background Is Related to Receiving Care and Using Services], Tampere: University of Tampere.

Van Aerschot, L., Mathew Puthenparambil, J., Olakivi, A. and Kröger, T. (2021) 'Psychophysical burden and lack of support: Reasons for care workers' intentions to leave their work in the Nordic countries', *International Journal of Social Welfare*, early view, https://doi.org/10.1111/ijsw.12520.

Van Houtven, C., Coe, N. and Skira, M. (2013) 'The effect of informal care on work and wages', *Journal of Health Economics*, vol 32, no 1, pp 240–52, doi:10.1016/j.jhealeco.2012.10.006.

van der Zwan, N. (2014) 'Making sense of financialization', *Socio-Economic Review*, vol 12, no 1, pp 99–129, doi:10.1093/ser/mwt020.

Vartiainen, P. (2019) *Filippiiniläisten sairaanhoitajien polut Suomeen: Tutkimus oppimisesta ja työyhteisöintegraatiosta kansainvälisen rekrytoinnin kontekstissa* [The Paths of Filipino Nurses to Finland: A Study on Learning and Integration Processes in the Context of International Recruitment], Tampere: University of Tampere.

Virokannas, E., Liuski, S. and Kuronen, M. (2018) 'The contested concept of vulnerability – A literature review', *European Journal of Social Work*, vol 23, no 2, pp 327–39, doi:10.1080/13691457.2018.1508001.

Virtanen, A. (2018) *Terveys- ja sosiaalipalvelujen henkilöstö 2014. Tilastoraportti 1/2018* [Health Care and the Social Welfare Personnel 2014. Statistical Report 1/2018], Helsinki: Finnish Institute for Health and Welfare.

Vitaliano, P. P., Zhang, J. and Scanlan, J. M. (2003) 'Is caregiving hazardous to one's physical health? A meta-analysis', *Psychological Bulletin*, vol 129, no 6, pp 946–72, doi:10.1037/0033-2909.129.6.946.

Vogl, J. (2017) *The Ascendancy of Finance*, Hoboken: John Wiley & Sons.

Voionmaa, V. (1929) *Tampereen historia. Osa II* [History of the City of Tampere. Part II]. Tampere: The City Tampere.

VTKL (2019) *Independent Preparedness for a Good Old Age 2018–2020.* VTKL, The Finnish Association for the Welfare of Older People, https://vtkl.fi/wp-content/uploads/2019/06/Prepare_for_old_age_project_brochure.pdf [accessed 24 April 2020].

Wærness, K. (1984) 'Caring as women's work in the welfare state' in H. Holter (ed) *Patriarchy in a Welfare State*, Oslo: Universitetsforlaget, pp 67–87.

Wærness, K. and Ringen, S. (1987) *Women in the Welfare State: The Case of Formal and Informal Old-age Care*, Stockholm: Swedish Institute for Social Research.

Wagner, D. (2005) *The Poorhouse. America's Forgotten Institution*, Lanham: Rowman & Littlefield.

Walker, A. (1984) 'The political economy of privatisation' in J. Le Grand and R. Robinson (eds) *Privatisation and the Welfare State*, London: Macmillan, pp 19–44.

Walkerdine, V. (2011) 'Shame on you! Intergenerational trauma and working class femininity on reality TV' in H. Wood and B. Skeggs (eds) *Reality Television and Class*, London: Palgrave Macmillan, pp 225–36.

Ward, L., Ray, M. and Tanner, D. (2020) 'Understanding the social care crisis in England through older people's lived experiences' in P. Urban and L. Ward (eds) *Care Ethics, Democratic Citizenship and the State. International Political Theory*, Cham: Palgrave Macmillan, pp 219–39.

Wiggan, J. (2012) 'Telling stories of 21st century welfare: The UK Coalition Government and the neo-liberal discourse of worklessness and dependency', *Critical Social Policy*, vol 32, no 3, pp 383-405, doi:10.1177/0261018312444413.

Williams, F. (2018) 'Care: Intersections of scales, inequalities and crises', *Current Sociology*, vol 66, no 4, pp 547-61, doi:10.1177/0011392118765206.

Wilson, E. (1977) *Women and the Welfare State*, London: Tavistock Publications.

Wrede, S. and Näre, L. (2013) 'Glocalising care in the Nordic countries', *Nordic Journal of Migration Research*, vol 3, no 2, pp 57–62.

Wrede, S., Henriksson, L., Høst, H., Johansson, S. and Dybbroe, B. (eds) (2008) *Care Work in Crisis. Reclaiming the Nordic Ethos of Care*, Lund: Studentlitteratur.

Wrede, S., Näre, L., Olakivi, A. and Nordberg, C. (2020) 'Neoliberal "flexibility" and the discursive incorporation of migrant labour in public eldercare in Finland' in N. Piper and C. Mora (eds) *The Palgrave Handbook of Gender and Migration: Global Perspectives*, London: Palgrave Macmillan, pp 253–68.

Yeandle, S., Kröger, T. and Cass, B. (2012) 'Voice and choice for users and carers? Developments in patterns of care for older people in Australia, England and Finland', *Journal of European Social Policy*, vol 22, no 4, pp 432–45, doi:10.1177/0958928712449775.

Yeates, N. (2009) *Globalizing Care Economies and Migrant Workers: Explorations in Global Care Chains*, London: Palgrave Macmillan.

Zechner, M. (2008) 'Care of older persons in transnational settings', *Journal of Aging Studies*, vol 22, no 1, pp 32–44, doi:10.1016/j.jaging.2007.02.002.

Zechner, M. (2017) 'Vastuutetut omaishoitajat markkinoilla' [Responsibilized informal carers in the markets of care], *Gerontologia*, vol 31, no 3, pp 179–94, doi:10.23989/gerontologia.63339.

Zechner, M. (2022) 'Economisation of care for older adults' in R. Baikady, S. M. Sajid, J. Przeperski, V. Nadesan, I. Rezaul and J. Gao (eds) *The Palgrave Handbook of Global Social Problems*, London: Palgrave, doi.org/10.1007/978-3-030-68127-2_300-1.

Zechner, M. and Anttonen, A. (2022) 'Care as work' in C. Ranci and T. Rostgaard (eds) *Research Handbook of Social Care Policy*, Cheltenham: Edward Elgar.

Zigante, V. (2018) *Informal Care in Europe. Exploring Formalisation, Availability and Quality*, Brussels: European Commission, https://data.europa.eu/doi/10.2767/78836 [accessed 2 May 2022].

Index

Printed and bound by CPI Group (UK) Ltd, Croydon, CR0 4YY

27/10/2024

14580557-0001